PRAISE FOR
OPTIMIZE YOUR IMMUNE SYSTEM

A treasure trove of practical information arriving at such a time of global urgency to strengthen our immune systems. The strong message throughout the book is the power of nutrition with various foods, nutrients and dietary supplements that are proven to be involved in preventing different diseases and minimizing pathophysiology of the disease. We can all have knowledge of the first line of defense for early interventions for our family's health and reduce the risk of more serious disease.

Diana Noland, MPH, RD, CCN, IFMCP, LD
founder of Noland Nutrition,
Co-Editor, *Integrative and Functional Medical Nutrition Therapy*

It is with great pleasure that I endorse and highly recommend Marie Ruggles's *Optimize Your Immune System.* It's an excellent, comprehensive guide to maximizing one's immune potential through nutrition and lifestyle modifications. Rarely do I review books with this level of guidance and step-by-step recommendations that can help individuals at every stage of readiness-for-change.

John Bagnulo, MPH, PhD

A nourishing read for all of us concerned about nutrition and immunity! This beautifully written book is a clear, actionable guide that delivers practical food-as-medicine and lifestyle strategies to bolster your immune defense. This is a wonderful and timely book!

Kathie Swift, MS, RDN
Co-Founder, Integrative and Functional Nutrition Academy
Author, *The Swift Diet*

If you want to take back control of your health, read this book. The section called *Immunity on a Budget* is a holy grail guide to an easy and affordable path to a stronger immune system.

Sabina Fasano
Founder, Solutions for Women

Optimize Your Immune System is chock-full of great information! The author, Marie Ruggles, masterfully wrote in a way that can be appreciated by those who already have some knowledge of the topic but want to take it to the next level, while also being easily understood by those who are just entering into this new way to approach wellness. The extensive detail is wonderful without being intimidating. A real "go to," at the ready at all times!

Veronica Anderson, RN, IAC

I always find Marie Ruggles's writing soothing, which complements her very relevant information on medical nutrition therapy and natural wellness. I highly recommend everyone from healthcare practitioners to everyday laypeople to read this straight-forward book. It will change their lives, help others, and provide solace when implementing Marie's recommendations. Her guidance will help support the body's immune system regardless of if or when we experience another pandemic—we all need to be prepared.

Diana L. Malkin-Washeim, PhD, MPH, RD, CDCES, CD-N
Director, Nutrition and Diabetes Program
BronxCare Diabetes Center of Excellence

Giving the consumer the ability to build their wellness right in the comfort of his or her own home is powerful! I know this will be a resource I will return to again and again.

Julie Mayring, PhD
Licensed Psychologist and Middle School Educator

Optimize Your Immune System

OPTIMIZE YOUR IMMUNE SYSTEM

Create Health and Resilience with a Kitchen Pharmacy

by

MARIE RUGGLES, RD, CN

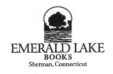

EMERALD LAKE
BOOKS
Sherman, Connecticut

Library of Congress Cataloging-in-Publication Data

Names: Ruggles, Marie, author.

Title: Optimize your immune system : create health and resilience with a

kitchen pharmacy / by Marie Ruggles.

Description: Sherman, CT : Emerald Lake Books, [2020] | Includes

bibliographical references and index. | Summary: "Many people think that

it's normal to come down with an illness each year and, for some, two or

three times a year. Yet researchers have scientifically proven that

nutrition and lifestyle factors can boost your immune system. Learn how

to build a kitchen pharmacy of whole foods, superfoods and nutrients to

provide a stable foundation for your health. And, when you're at an

increased risk of infection, know what to do to derail a virus before it

takes hold. Follow this immune-boosting roadmap to be healthier and less

prone to viral infections"-- Provided by publisher.

Identifiers: LCCN 2020027826 (print) | LCCN 2020027827 (ebook) | ISBN

9781945847301 (trade paperback) | ISBN 9781945847318 (epub)

Subjects: LCSH: Natural immunity. | Nutrition. | Health. | Immune system.

Classification: LCC QR185.2 .R84 2020 (print) | LCC QR185.2 (ebook) | DDC

616.07/9--dc23

LC record available at https://lccn.loc.gov/2020027826

LC ebook record available at https://lccn.loc.gov/2020027827

This book is dedicated to my husband, Shelly,
who was a primary champion of this work.
His support has kept me energized to finally
bring it to completion.

This book is also dedicated to you, my dear reader.
You are the reason I approach each day
with a passion for learning and teaching.
My prayer is that you will be strong and healthy
so you can walk in your purpose.

Disclaimer and Important Safety Notes

All recommendations are for non-pregnant, non-nursing adults. The contents of this book are for educational purposes only. It should not be used in any way as a substitute for professional medical advice or treatment with your physician or other qualified healthcare provider. It is not provided to diagnose, prescribe or treat any condition. All recommendations are for general guidance only and do not include all available information on nutritional immunity. The information is for strengthening the immune system and not treatment or diagnosis of any sickness. Every foreign invader has unique characteristics and may respond in a manner that differs from the activity demonstrated in the research. Since every person has a unique physiology and responds differently, you should consult your primary physician or qualified healthcare provider prior to using any new food or product. Supporting one's immune system is in no way a guarantee against any illness.

There is no assumed responsibility or liability for errors, inaccuracies or omissions in this content. Neither the author nor the publisher warrants that any information contained within is fully complete and they shall have neither liability nor responsibility to any person or entity with respect to any loss or damage caused or alleged to be caused directly or indirectly by this book, nor do we make any claims or promises of your ability to be well. When considering the use of supplements, follow the directions of your physician or qualified healthcare provider.

Be advised that links contained in this book may be affiliate links and the author may earn a commission if you use them to buy products or services mentioned in this book. This is at no additional cost to you, and the author has only recommended items she truly believes are beneficial. However, the author and publisher disclaim any liability that may result from your involvement with any such websites or products. You should perform your own due diligence before buying any mentioned products or services.

CONTENTS

INTRODUCTION

This is a book about wellness. Supporting the crucial function of your immune system is one of the best things you can do to maintain your health; it is your first line of defense. Everything you eat and drink either strengthens or weakens your immune system.

Start with your food. I'm going to show you how to transform a corner of your pantry into a kitchen pharmacy, stocked with healing foods, teas, spices and supplements to ensure you have immune-optimizing solutions within reach when your system needs a boost. This is known as the "food-as-medicine" approach to health, and it is backed by thousands of clinical research studies.

I started my career in research and continue to be impressed with the expansion of clinical studies in nutritional immunology. Every day, new clinical trials are revealing the immune-enhancing effects of specific foods and nutrients. My mission is to take the science out of the lab and bring it into your kitchen in simple, actionable steps.

You will learn how to build a strong foundation. This will help you to experience a better outcome, no matter what immune challenge you are facing. In addition to preventive health and overall wellness, there will be a focus on viral infections,[1] including what to do when you have been in an unhealthy environment or when you are starting to feel like something is coming on. In a nutshell, you're

---

1   Colds, the flu and other conditions with similar respiratory symptoms are usually caused by a virus.

going to learn how to get ahead of a virus; bolstering your defenses *before* it gets ugly.

Typically, you feel fine for a few days while a virus is busy spreading. It's only when the viral load significantly increases that you develop the symptoms that let you know you are sick. Soon after one virus passes through, it's replaced by another one or some other threat to your health. That's why I suggest starting with building a foundation that will strengthen and prepare your immune system for whatever comes at it.

The information provided in this book is for maintaining wellness, not for the treatment of illness or a specific virus. Each virus has a unique biology and requires different interventions. The best way to increase your chance for a successful outcome is by using a variety of immune-boosting supports that offer unique benefits. This approach allows you to cover all the bases by optimizing your internal defense system.

More on that later. For now, let's talk about what happens when you go to a party.

Some of those people you are hugging and kissing are coming down with something, but they don't know it yet. People who are carrying a virus often feel fine for the initial two to five days (or longer) while it's in their body setting up house and multiplying. Yup. Your friends are out partying while their systems are being overtaken. It's not until the virus reaches mass multiplication after several days that their symptoms keep them home. We call these people "shedders." They are passing the virus on to others, often without any awareness of their own infectious state.

Meanwhile, you're shaking hands and sharing the same wine bottle, using the same serving spoons, and then scratching your nose with that hand. You're also breathing the same air that may carry droplets (with invisible uninvited microorganisms) right into your lungs. It's the same scenario when you place your hands on the grocery cart handle, bathroom faucet or equipment at the gym. Some germs can survive for longer than ten hours on a surface.

And guess what? When someone who is fifteen feet away from you sneezes, you're in their water droplet zone!

Taking deliberate action to strengthen your immune system is the first step in staying healthy along with handwashing and other baseline hygiene precautions. When I think of my immune system, the image that comes to me is a group of guards at the door who decide who gets in, who can stay and, most important, who gets deleted from the party list!

That's what this book is all about; creating a high-functioning immune system with the crucial foods and nutrients to keep you well all year long. In times when additional support is needed on a short-term basis, further immune resilience can be achieved by using natural reinforcements.

By paying daily attention to nourishing this system of defense, your entire body will benefit. What's good for the immune system is also good for the rest of your body, from your brain to the appearance of your skin. A robust immune system will help protect you from autoimmune conditions, such as arthritis, cancer and many other unwanted guests.

Optimizing immune function is the first step to providing an internal shield of protection and enjoying better health all year long. The three steps for optimization include:

1. **Act Now.** This is the time to prepare your immune system for the season ahead. Give your body some TLC (or "tender loving care") every day. Being proactive is key.

2. **Be Ready**. Keep a few natural wellness options on hand for when you need to step it up a notch to support your immune system after being near a sick person or in an unhealthy environment.

3. **Take Control**. Take back your power, knowing you can strengthen your internal defense system with food, supplements and healthy lifestyle choices.

This book will show you exactly how to accomplish each of these three steps.

My background is in nutrition and public health, and I am a certified diabetes educator. My experience includes over forty years in the wellness arena. I have found that staying well requires more than a healthy diet. This led me to incorporate a variety of simple, natural wellness strategies and products into my programs with tremendous success. While there are many immunity-strengthening supplements available, the ones you will find here are primarily food-based, including powerful extracts of elderberries and grapefruit seeds. These help me to keep it simple with confidence, knowing they deliver. And I just love everything "food." I hope you will also gain the same appreciation.

These are not your only options. They are what my work has focused on. There are other approaches including herbs, naturopathic and traditional Chinese wellness strategies that also have much to offer. What I'm sharing here is easy to find and simple to use; a treasure trove of wellness you can implement on your own. As new clinical trials emerge, additional information for optimizing immune support will become available. Feel free to consult other natural practitioners along the way to further enhance your wellness.

You are the owner of an inner army responsible for protection, maintenance and renewal. This is your personal "homeland security" system, which needs reinforcements for optimal function. The key to optimizing your security system is knowing when to take extra measures to strengthen your innate disease and virus-fighting immune system. The innate immune system includes your first line of soldiers to enter battle. These early risers are critical in controlling the escalation of conflict—the multiplication of viruses. In this book, you will learn how to activate this system for optimal results.

If you are wondering whether there is solid scientific evidence on the role of nutrition and immunity, check out the U.S. government's research database at PubMed.gov. There is a very robust body of research demonstrating the undeniable role food and nutrients play in strengthening immune resilience.

Simply typing "vitamins and infection" into the search bar of the PubMed database will show over 25,000 studies on this topic, with more being added every week. More specific searches, like "zinc and virus" or "pneumonia and nutrition" each bring up more than 4,000 studies. While searching for "probiotics and infection" yields over 7,000 results.

With a growing interest in viral immunity and the existing body of data showing the essential role of nutrition in immune resilience, these numbers are bound to increase dramatically over the next few years. In this book, I interpret the science for you in a way that makes it easy to translate into what to serve for dinner.

You will also learn how to develop a simple home inventory of natural wellness options. Choose those that fit *your* lifestyle. These options include whole foods, superfoods, spices, vitamins D and C (plus other critical nutrients and supplements), teas, mood management, sleep, activity and immune-support supplements.

Superfoods are foods that contain special therapeutic compounds, also known as "bioactives." I like the way Amanda Archibald, RD, author of *The Genomic Kitchen* describes bioactives.

> ...bioactives function like a switch that, when activated, sets in motion a series of biochemical steps, akin to knocking over a series of dominos. The result of this cascade is the activation of certain genes.

I believe God designed your amazing body with innate wisdom for knowing exactly what to do. The support offered in this book is derived from God's creation (plants). Including these reinforcements maximizes your body's efforts to efficiently carry out the job your creator designed it to do. Extra support is often needed because of a lifestyle that may include unhealthy food choices, chronic distress and toxin overload.

I am going to provide specific steps for developing your own home inventory of natural wellness options. When specific items are mentioned (teas, supplements, foods, etc.), I will provide guidance on which brands and products I use and recommend to my students. These suggestions are highlighted as "Products I Love," some of which may already be found in your kitchen. Whenever possible, I suggest a few products, simply to give you some price options.

When I recommend brands, it's to guide you to "safe" companies, meaning they don't use unnecessary fillers, which can be a source of contaminants. Their capsules contain exactly what is listed on the label. It also means the company has been thoughtful about the sourcing of ingredients. This is not the case with all brands.

My recommendations represent just a sample of the many excellent nutraceutical supplement brands. Feel free to "price shop" using these guidelines to review other products.

For a continuously updated list of products I love, visit my website at marieruggles.com/products.

The body has many wellness maintenance management systems we could talk about. The immune system is a great starting place. Even if your primary area of focus may be on another system, you will still benefit from the immune system focus. You can always layer on targeted support for your personal area of concern. True wellness begins with addressing core imbalances that, when brought into balance, will correct many areas of your physiology, strength, cognition, mood and resilience. In "Medical Resources" on page 122, I have provided a list of nutrition-minded and natural medicine practitioners who can further assist in your wellness journey.

Why am I so excited to share this strategy for optimizing immune function and getting ahead of a virus with you? There is truly no need to dread being plagued with unhealthy winter days or everyday health challenges. This is because you can take care of your body all year long, creating strength and resilience. With a bit of information, you will understand how to get back into the driver's seat. More on that in Chapter 1. Immune System 101, where you will learn how you may be unintentionally blocking your immune system's vital activities.

What tools do you need? Choose whatever resonates with you. Start with what's accessible and easy. In Chapter 2. Foods that Optimize Immune Function, I will introduce you to some very surprising foods that contain bioactive compounds that deeply nourish your cells, calm inflammation, and fortify the immune response. Some of these might be readily available in your kitchen. You will find easy ideas for incorporating my strategies into your day with my "Whole Foods Quick Start Guide." Whole foods are the cornerstone of vibrant health.

I have made every effort to address various topics in this book in a way that's easy to understand. When you understand the concepts, you're more likely to be motivated to consistently follow through on my recommendations.

You will also learn there are certain foods that can hinder immune function. Too much sugar, for example, can derail immune activity. The same is true with stress, physical activity and sleep. Each of these is a factor you can modify yourself, putting you into the driver's seat of your own wellness.

An adequate supply of nutrients is another one of the key reinforcements for priming your immune system to be on constant surveillance and to mount a vigorous attack when needed. In Chapter 3. Superfoods That Optimize Gut Health & Immune Function and Chapter 4. Nutrients and Supplements That Optimize Immune Function, you will learn about superfoods and specific nutrients that strengthen your immune system.

According to Diana Noland, MPH, RDN, IFMCP, LD, a pioneer in the field of clinical nutrition and co-editor of *Integrative and Functional Medical Nutrition Therapy*:

> It is now recognized that an individual's vulnerability to infection is associated with nutrition status. Nutrients maintain the integrity of the immune system.

The critical interplay between sleep, exercise and mood, as well as the function of your immune system will be addressed in Chapter 5. Lifestyle Factors That Affect Immune Function. In Chapter 6. Putting It All Together, you will find a simple, reference summary for self-care. This is where you will see what it looks like to put my recommendations into practice during each phase, including daily wellness, exposure to an unhealthy person or environment, and the need for extra immune support when you feel like something is coming on.

Can you picture your family having great health all year long? My *most* favorite part of teaching others about having a home inventory of natural wellness options is sharing the message that you can *take back your power*. If anyone in my family wakes up with something going on, I typically have a safe and simple option to take care of it, so there are fewer missed days of school, work and play!

Taking back your power is like having boots on the ground in your own home. I always feel confidently equipped to take care of myself and my loved ones. My hope for you after reading this book is that you will feel more empowered and less victimized by circumstances. We regularly take actions to protect ourselves and loved ones from harm. This may include the use of protective equipment, like seat belts and biking helmets, or the scheduling of periodic dental appointments, but do you ever think about actively protecting your immune system?

I hope you will embrace personal responsibility for the care and keeping of your immune system, knowing that wellness starts when your feet hit the floor every morning. If you are well all winter, it's in part because of what you did during the other eight months of the year. Are you already starting to feel the power?

I encourage you to read the entire book to get a feel for the wellness options that are literally at your fingertips. Then, keep the book handy to serve as a reference guide, which is where Chapter 6. Putting It All Together will come in handy. After all, you are a busy person. No need to memorize anything; the information is in here. Keep this reference in the kitchen or other convenient location. I wrote this book and yet I still refer to it for guidance!

There you have it. After putting my tips into practice, your personal security system will be charged and ready. Know that as you read, I will be in prayer for you, hoping each chapter will shower your home with the wellness blessings you most need at this time.

CHAPTER 1. IMMUNE SYSTEM 101

The immune system's prime function is to protect your body. Knowing some basic information about how your immune system works will go a long way in helping you to take better care of it and your entire body. This extra care will pay it forward with big health dividends through all seasons and as you age.

In addition to the daily and seasonal challenges your immune system is actively confronting, it is a key player in preventing potential ailments. Every day, this system is busy targeting radical cells for destruction and neutralizing the daily onslaught of toxins. For all these reasons, keeping your immune system strong and ready to fight should be a top priority.

White blood cells are one of the key components of your immune system responsible for surveillance and defense. There are several varieties of white blood cells, each with specialized jobs. For simplicity, we are going to group their overall mission into:

- Attack
- Engulf
- Digest

Other components of your immune system are equally important and have specific jobs. They are all warrior cells. Some fight parasites, produce fighter chemicals, or develop antibodies. These components of your immune system are continuously at work. In times of high demand, the workload is increased along with the need for more fuel.

The fuel that drives these activities comes in the form of vitamins and minerals. Immune cells love nutrients. They even have receptor sites for them. Cell receptor sites are like parking spaces. Your immune cells have parking spaces with the names of specific nutrients on them. Taking good care of your body all year long by supplying it with a continuous store of nutrients will give your body a reserve to draw upon in times of increased demand.

Your immune system will thank you for the extra care and attention by:

1. Increasing the number of immune cells and defense compounds.
2. Strengthening the barriers, including your skin, gut bacteria and the mucous membranes of your nose, throat, airways and lungs.
3. Enhancing the activity of immune cells, including detoxification, maintenance, renewal and killing off foreign invaders, such as viruses.
4. Blocking attachment of invaders.
5. Managing inflammation.
6. Working harder and longer to remove debris from degraded cells and toxins.

When it comes to viruses, your immune system can intervene at any stage of an invasion. Intervention might take place at the "wall," which is where the barriers, such as mucous membranes, stand guard. If the virus does gain entry, your warrior cells may prevent it from attaching onto a cell in your sinuses or lungs. And if the virus has successfully evaded the barriers and entered a cell, your immune killer cells can disable its ability to replicate and spread to other nearby cells.

With the understanding of how important supporting the immune system is, its optimal function starts with your daily self-care habits, including healthy foods, exercise, hydration, quality sleep, mood management and providing an adequate supply of nutrients and bioactives. It can take months to reboot your immune system, or longer if you have really been "off the trail." Now is the time to start, keeping in mind that today's healthy habits will protect you in the upcoming seasons.

Your immune system is a remarkably designed army of combatant cells that work at maximum efficiency when you:

1. Nourish it.
2. Avoid immunotoxicity.
3. Provide well-timed reinforcements.
4. Avoid blockages that disrupt your immune system's activity.

To nourish your immune system, you must provide a daily supply of vitamins, minerals and other bioactive compounds that are essential ingredients for driving immune activity. This is something you can do today to ramp up for those times when your system has an increased need for protection, such as defeating foreign invaders.

You can avoid immunotoxicity by replacing toxic cleaners, air fresheners, processed foods, candles, shampoos, moisturizers, toothpastes and other personal care products that flood your cells with chemicals that block normal functioning.

As for providing well-timed reinforcements, let's look at what happens when unhealthy organisms enter your body. According to Aristo Vojdani, PhD, microbiologist and immunologist, pathogen activity can be described with the acronym IRS: Infection, Replication and Spread. In a healthy person, the immune system is instantly alerted and begins to deploy killer cells to take out the enemy. Sometimes, unbeknownst to you, the unhealthy organisms find a way to quietly evade the killer cells and start to multiply. For this reason, it's critical to act as soon as possible. During this time, you feel fine. After two to five days (or longer) of multiplication, you start to recognize you need immune support because you now have uncomfortable symptoms.

The best time to act is before you are in distress so your immune system is ready for any challenge. The second best time is as soon as you have been with an unhealthy person, in an unhealthy environment, or have a weakened immune system from stress, grief or depression. On a personal note, I am most vulnerable to infection when my stress level is high or when I'm burning the candle at both ends. These two scenarios often occur simultaneously, creating a double whammy.

When your body gives a signal (fatigue, scratchy throat, slight congestion), it's an alert that it's time to act. Acting immediately will pay off tremendously. This is your opportunity to bring in the reinforcements—superfoods and immune-enhancing supplements.

It is crucial to avoid blockages that disrupt your immune system's activity. The way we live can inhibit your immune system's performance, even as sophisticated as it is.

Toxins can be found in our environment as well as in products we use and foods we ingest. Unfortunately, these toxins can block our body's ability to protect and renew itself with precision (as it is intended to do), thereby derailing the healing powers of the immune system. They can be found in the air, as pesticides on the food we eat, in processed foods, and contaminants from food containers. They can even be found in the chemicals used to manufacture cleaning and personal care products.

Sugar can also sabotage your immune system. Additionally, toxic emotions are also top saboteurs of a resilient inner-defense system.

Sixty years ago, toxins started to enter our environment in massive amounts. According to Joseph Pizzorno, ND, Author of *The Toxin Solution: How Hidden Poisons in the Air, Water, Food and Products We Use Are Destroying Our Health*, "Toxins are now the invisible primary drivers of countless health problems. They block normal immune function and disrupt every aspect of our physiology," and this has been shown repeatedly in cutting-edge research.

Daily use of chemical-laden products creates a virtual cesspool of toxins in your body that block optimal immune function. Your body has an innate capacity to detox, but was not designed to manage the current level of toxic exposure most of us experience.

The good news is there are many easy steps you can take today to decrease toxin exposure. Swapping out toxic products for chemical-free cleaning and personal care products is one way to immediately stop the daily influx of damaging compounds.

Start by checking the labels of your cleaning or personal care products. Type any name you don't recognize into Google preceded by the phrase "dangers of" and see what comes up.

I once assumed products on the store shelf were safe. How could they be there otherwise? I also assumed the government oversees product safety. Not so. The government requires no pre-market testing. The FDA lets the cosmetics industry self-police, which leaves the public vulnerable to toxicity.

According to the Environmental Working Group:

> The Food and Drug Administration has no authority to require companies to test cosmetic products for safety and the agency does not review or approve most ingredients before they go on the market; companies may use any ingredient in their products without approval. In the past 30 years, the FDA has banned only 11 ingredients from use in personal care products, whereas the European Union has banned more than 1,000. The average woman uses up to fifteen personal care products daily, exposing herself on average to 126 daily toxins.

Which products should you consider swapping out for safer alternatives? Consider the cleaning products you use, as well as your daily personal care items, including shampoo, toothpaste and moisturizer. Remember, when you choose natural immune-support options, you are also likely avoiding chemical-laden alternatives.

Also, consider the packaging choices you make. When you eat canned soup or drink water from a plastic bottle, your blood levels of BPA and other plastics increase dramatically. To find out more about the toxins in the packaging you use, contact food manufacturers for information about the content of their packaging. Eden is the only company in the United States I know of that does not use harmful chemicals in the lining of their cans.

According to the Environmental Working Group:

> ...in order to receive organic certification, packaged foods must not only be free of toxic pesticides but also of thousands of added chemicals like artificial preservatives, colors and flavors. Only 40 synthetic substances have been approved for organic packaged foods. By contrast, thousands of chemicals can be added to conventional packaged foods, many of which don't require independent government approval for use.

This is another reason to go organic as much as possible. Choosing organic options will also go a long way to help you avoid another chemical, glyphosate. This toxin is considered to be a probable human carcinogen. According to the World Health Organization, glyphosate is found in many foods we consume daily, such as nonorganic oats (including granola and oat-based cereals), pasta, crackers, pizza and ice cream.

The job of your immune system is to target and destroy unhealthy microbes, such as viruses and bacteria. It will work much better when blockages caused by toxins in our system are removed. These blockages can overwhelm your defenses or impede immune cell activity by preventing the entry of key compounds into your cells.

Remember, you will need the highest levels of support from your immune system at times when you are in emotional distress. Stress will sabotage your immune defenses. Yet, this is the time we are most likely to let our guard down and stop taking care of ourselves. Don't make this big mistake. The times when you are stressed out and experiencing challenges are the times when you need to step up your game. Being proactive against stress is essential for ensuring your immune system is well-equipped to launch a well-fortified defense to protect you.

CHAPTER 2. FOODS THAT OPTIMIZE IMMUNE FUNCTION

L et's start building the foundation of wellness by focusing on the basic ingredients your immune system needs to run effectively. Nutrient deficiencies compromise immune function. Supplements play an important role, but food should always be your primary source of nourishment. Every bite of food will either nourish your cells or damage them. Fueling your body with a daily banquet of nutrient-rich whole foods, including a variety of vegetables, will impact every aspect of how well your entire body functions. Attending to your health daily will affect how your body responds to wellness challenges. Nutrients play a critical role in priming your system, activating immune cells, and building resilience. Plant foods have been shown in clinical trials to improve resistance to viral infection. Following the suggestions in this chapter will kick-start your kitchen pharmacy and provide your body with a solid foundation for health.

As important as eating healthy is, don't feel as if you must do everything right away. Start with whatever is easiest for you and continue to expand your wellness routine at a pace that works for you. I'm hoping to engage you in the bigger (and more rewarding) picture of a long-term lifestyle of daily wellness habits, not a quick unsustainable fix. Habits can be little acts grown over time, ultimately changing the makeup of your body for enhanced wellness from head to toe.

Keep this book in a convenient location so you can refer to it whenever needed. Most importantly, don't stress. After all, stress depletes your immune system!

Whole Foods Nutrition

THE FIRST STEP TO STRENGTHENING immunity is to swap out processed foods for whole foods. This transition may take some time to accomplish. That's okay. Every step along the way, your cells will be thanking you. You will learn how to make delicious meals, have more energy, and look healthier. In addition, the appearance of your skin may noticeably improve. It's hard to appreciate the issues you're preventing, but some problems that were brewing simply won't arise because you have steered your metabolism onto a new track. You will be changing your constitution, deleting the junk, and fueling your cells with the bioactives they are craving. Your mind and mood will improve, and you will be working toward cancer prevention with your fork. For now, be easy on yourself and your family. Enjoy your gradual transition by experimenting with tasty recipes that nourish and renew your body.

Notice I said gradual. I really want you to start slowly as you move into a healthier place. I didn't change my eating pattern the day I earned my nutrition degree. Far from it! It has been a process. Truthfully, my eating strategy continues to be tweaked as new research emerges. Start with replacing one item. If you're cooking for others, expect resistance. That's okay and perfectly normal. Continue to experiment. Be respectful of their need for the familiar, but be creative with your transition process.

Your immune system relies upon a continuous supply of hydration, vitamins, minerals and other bioactive compounds for efficient functioning. All of these supplies can be found in whole foods and are the drivers of your immune system's white (killer) cells' activity. Conversely, processed foods derail cell function, sabotaging your body's ability to consistently activate an effective program of defense.

Whole foods, on the other hand, are in their natural state. They provide fiber, enzymes, prebiotics, probiotics, essential fats, proteins, vitamins, minerals and many other important bioactives. Fresh ingredients that are in season are the best choices. Whole organic foods contain only the ingredients found in nature. These nutrients direct all aspects of your metabolism. Nutritionists often refer to this bounty of nutrients as containing the "innate intelligence" our bodies need for optimal functioning.

If you can buy local produce at the store or farmers' market, that's even better. It will be fresher, which means more nutrients. Plus, who doesn't love a weekend trip to the farmers' market? Nothing beats a fresh stock of local fruits and veggies while supporting your neighborhood farmers.

Consuming processed or convenience food deprives your body of essential nutrients. They typically also deliver a bevy of toxic non-food ingredients. Over time, this will negatively affect your appearance, energy, mood and overall health. Therefore, the goal is to saturate your cells with a consistent supply of nutrients by choosing whole foods, including an abundance of plant food choices. So, what are plant foods? Vegetables, fruits, nuts, seeds and legumes (beans).

Many processed foods are compromised by the addition of artificial colors, flavors, chemical preservatives, artificial sweeteners, excess refined salt and sugar. Processing results in loss of vital nutrients. While many of the processed food choices are fortified with synthetic vitamins, it is not an adequate substitute. Added vitamins may replace a minor portion of nutrients, but none of the other essential bioactives.

To make matters worse, containers of these convenience foods, such as microwave popcorn, often contain chemicals that leach into the food. Plastic coatings and containers also leach toxic particles, which can be further exacerbated when heated up in a microwave. As mentioned in Chapter 1, these toxins derail immune activity.

There is a place for minimally processed foods, such as pre-chopped vegetables, applesauce, tomato sauce, oatmeal, canned salmon and beans. For example, cacao beans—a very nutritious food—need to be processed into a cocoa powder to be used in cooking. What I'm referring to here are the highly processed convenience foods that often have long ingredient lists. Yes, these foods can make for easy kitchen prep, but the price may be a profound effect on your health. This has been borne out in hundreds of research studies and is something nutritionists witness every day in clinical practice.

These processed foods can deprive children whose families rely on convenience and fast foods of essential life skills, like learning cooking skills, the satisfying teamwork involved in putting together a family meal, and the soul nourishment of consuming a meal prepared with love. The failure to build a robust immune defense early in life may ultimately be seen later in the form of various wellness challenges—physical, emotional and cognitive. To this day, my kids still thank me for establishing a sense of pride and enjoyment for cooking at home and preparing something that both tastes good and is healthy.

After forty years of converting thousands of others to a plant-strong, whole foods eating pattern, I can assure you people following this strategy have more energy, fewer cravings and better sleep. They simply feel better.

A recent study in the *American Journal of Clinical Nutrition* found that fruits and vegetables decrease inflammation and enhance the function of immune cells.[2] Don't worry, I'm not asking you to become a vegetarian. I am asking you to start replacing some meat meals with bean meals. Include at least a half plate of vegetables with all meals as a way of flooding your cells with the vital nourishment

---

2   Hosseini B, Berthon BS, Saedisomeolia A, et al. Effects of fruit and vegetable consumption on inflammatory biomarkers and immune cell populations: a systematic literature review and meta-analysis. *Am J Clin Nutr*. 2018; 108(1):136-155.

needed for optimizing immune function. This will decrease cell damage that accelerates the disease process and aging in general.

There are so many other reasons to go whole when it comes to your plate. Many studies, including a landmark study in the *British Medical Journal*, found that those who ate the most processed foods were more likely to have a stroke or heart disease. They reported that every 5% increase in processed foods led to a corresponding increase in the level of heart and blood vessel disease. Strokes occur when a blood vessel leading to the brain is blocked or torn. Research also indicates plant foods can dampen an overactive immune response, which may lead to increased uncomfortable symptoms and collateral damage during sickness.

Did I mention this is also the best aging-well strategy? Take good care of your body today and it will reward you tenfold as you age!

Finding Whole Food Recipes

Many bloggers provide a variety of good recipes. Type "top whole foods blogs" into your browser. Select two to follow and see if their style resonates with you. Check their websites for top-rated recipes. Continue this process until you locate a blog with appealing recipes that seem easy enough to make. Search for a Lentil Bolognese recipe for starters. Jazz it up with a little red pepper!

I have been following Vegan Richa, who features flavorful vegan fare, and the Minimalist Baker, who includes poultry recipes and keeps it simple. These are just two examples. I often mix it up with other bloggers.

Also, check out *The Flavor Bible* by Karen Page and Andrew Dornenburg for help with reinventing the way you flavor your foods. This book has transformed many kitchens, including mine.

Whole food recipes should contain generous amounts of vegetables. If this is new to you, be patient during the learning process. Your perseverance will pay off big time.

It may even open a whole new world of interesting conversation as following food bloggers is a hot topic!

Two simple ways to make healthy choices include reducing processed foods and increasing whole foods (and more meals that are truly home-cooked).

Step 1: Reduce Processed Foods

BECOME FAMILIAR WITH THESE so you can recognize them when shopping, planning meals, or eating on-the-run. Minimize your intake of these processed foods and ingredients:

- Agave
- Artificial sweeteners
- Bacon
- Bagels
- Candy
- Chicken nuggets
- Chips
- Convenience or deli meats (cold cuts, sausages, hot dogs)
- Corn syrup, including high-fructose corn syrup
- Donuts
- Fast food restaurants
- French fries
- Fried foods[3]
- Frozen appetizers
- Frozen meals
- Frozen vegetables doused in sauce
- Fruit-flavored beverages

---

3   Fried foods from restaurants are usually cooked in oil that has been used repeatedly. According to Paul Pitchford, author of *Healing with Whole Foods*, "This oil is the equivalent of ingesting car wax." Reusing frying oil creates compounds that are lethal to your cells.

- Fruit juice[4]
- Gravy and packaged sauces
- High-salt foods
- Instant oatmeal
- Instant Raman noodles and other packaged soup mixes
- Margarine or fake butter spreads
- Mashed potato flakes
- Meat substitutes
- Microwave popcorn
- Muffins
- Packaged and convenience foods
- Pastry
- Pie
- Pizza
- Prepared foods that have a long ingredient list or a lot of salt, sugar or preservatives
- Processed cheese (such as American cheese)
- Puffed low-carb snacks
- Refined cereals (most boxed cereals)
- Refined vegetable oils (soybean, canola, corn, sunflower, safflower, hydrogenated, shortening, trans fats and vegetable blends)
- Refrigerator rolls
- Roasted nuts[5]

---

4   When fruit is dried or processed into a juice, its fructose content is concentrated. Excess amounts of fructose are unhealthy. Limit fructose to 10 grams per meal or 25 grams per day. Other foods high in fructose include certain fruits, especially dried fruits, pancake syrup, soda and sweetened beverages, including cocktail mixes. Fresh berries, pineapple and citrus fruits are low-fructose choices. Dried fruits and deeply colored fruit juices are on the Whole Foods list, but with a note to only use in small amounts.

5   Roasting damages the oils in nuts. If not using them within one week, store nuts in the freezer to prevent their oils from going rancid.

- ᔍ Salad dressings made with canola, vegetable, corn, safflower or soybean oil (most restaurant dressings)[6]
- ᔍ Soda, including diet
- ᔍ Sweetened drinks
- ᔍ Vitamin-enhanced water
- ᔍ White flour and products made with enriched flour
- ᔍ White sugar

Step 2: Include More Whole Foods

THESE ARE WHOLE OR MINIMALLY processed foods that should replace as many processed foods as possible. Consider replacing meat and poultry meals with bean or legume meals, such as lentil soup, black bean burgers, bean and vegetable salad. Or try some of these other healthy options:

- ᔍ Alliums, such as onions, garlic, leeks, chives, scallions or shallots
- ᔍ Beans or legumes, all varieties (dry, canned[7] or frozen)
- ᔍ Beef, preferably grass-fed and organic[8]
- ᔍ Black-eyed peas (dried, canned or frozen)
- ᔍ Bone broth
- ᔍ Butter, ghee
- ᔍ Canned coconut milk
- ᔍ Canned fruit
- ᔍ Cheese (not processed types, like American cheese)
- ᔍ Lentils (dried or pre-cooked)
- ᔍ Deeply-colored fruit juices, such as pomegranate, tart cherry or concord grape[9]

---

6   Make your own dressing or purchase fat-free dressing and add extra virgin olive oil.

7   Preferably from Eden brand.

8   Avoid char-grilled, blackened meat. It increases the risk of cancer.

9   Only in small amounts; no more than 4 fl oz for an average-sized adult.

- Dried fruit[10]
- Eggs (preferably free-range)
- Fats and oils, including olive, avocado, coconut, pastured butter, ghee or flax (which should not be used with heat)
- Fresh fish[11]
- Fresh fruits
- Fresh vegetables
- Frozen fruit
- Frozen vegetables (plain)
- Ground flaxseeds[12]
- Hemp seeds[13]
- Hummus or bean dip
- Jarred artichokes[14]
- Jarred broth concentrates
- Jarred pesto
- Jarred roasted peppers
- Jarred sardines or salmon (canned works too)
- Jarred tomatoes or tomato sauce
- Microgreens
- Millet
- Miso paste (can be made with vegetables, rice, legumes or soy)
- Mushrooms
- Nuts and seeds (raw)[15]
- Nut butters[16]
- Nut milks

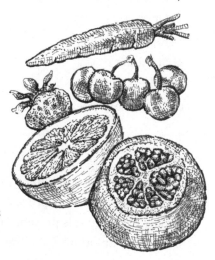

---

10 See footnote 9.
11 Choose low-mercury species of fish.
12 Store in freezer to prevent oxidation.
13 See footnote 12.
14 "Jarred" refers to glass containers, which help you to avoid the toxic plastic lining found in cans. Jarred fish may be hard to find or too expensive, so using canned is okay.
15 Store in freezer.
16 Store in refrigerator.

- ❧ Oats (old fashioned, extra thick or steel-cut oats or oat bran)
- ❧ Olives
- ❧ Poultry, preferably free-range and organic
- ❧ Rice (brown, red, black or basmati)[17]
- ❧ Quinoa
- ❧ Rice crackers
- ❧ Sorghum
- ❧ Tofu[18]
- ❧ Yogurt, unsweetened

A Note on Salt

There is a whole version of salt, often referred to as "sea salt." Whole salt is unprocessed and contains the natural balance of minerals present in the water it was harvested from. The amount of sodium it contains is in balance to the other minerals present in the salt. Authentic sea salt has a full complement of minerals, which provide additional flavor and essential nourishment for the healthy functioning of your cells. It doesn't contain any "anti-clumping" agents commonly added to regular table salt. True sea salt is never white, which indicates that the essential minerals have been washed out. The products I love are grey and pink in color, indicating the presence of healthy sea minerals.

Products I Love

♥ Selina Naturally Celtic Sea Salt

---

17 Many rice products have been found to be high in arsenic, a carcinogen. Try to purchase from companies such as Lundberg, who monitor the arsenic content of their products.

18 Purchase as much organic as possible. Soy should always be purchased organic since all nonorganic soy is GMO (genetically modified).

> ♥ Premier Research Labs Premier Pink Salt
> ♥ Selina Naturally Celtic Sea Salt Gourmet Seaweed Seasoning

Below you will find my Whole Foods Quick Start Guide, which will give you a good overview of what whole foods to eat at mealtime. Avoid any foods you cannot tolerate, since even some healthy foods may not be a good fit for the biology of your body.

Whole Foods Quick Start Guide

IN THE PAGES THAT FOLLOW, some foods will be listed by groups, such as vegetables, fruits and spices. Whenever an item could fit into multiple categories, the most common one is used for ease of reference. Therefore, a tomato, cucumber or pepper, while technically a fruit because it has seeds, will be listed according to its traditional placement as a vegetable. Many spices, like garlic, turmeric and ginger, are technically root vegetables, but you'll see them listed as spices instead.

If you'd like to download a copy of this guide, include a progress tracker so you can chart how well you're doing with eating the whole foods way, visit marieruggles.com/progress.

General Tips

DRINK TWO CUPS OF WATER during the first hour after waking to flush and hydrate. Do this before eating breakfast.

Eat fruits and vegetables from a variety of color groups throughout the day, including snacks.

As a general rule, have a half plate of vegetables at each meal or a minimum of five servings daily. Each serving doesn't need to be of different vegetables; large servings of three different vegetables will work. A large salad will provide at least two servings, and filling half your lunch and dinner plates with vegetables will get you to your goal.

Eat one to three fruits a day, unless you have an issue with fructose malabsorption, insulin resistance or blood sugar control. In which case, just eat more vegetable servings instead of fruit.

Vegetables can be prepared in many delicious ways. Explore recipes for creative ideas to highlight their flavors and expand upon your usual preparation techniques. There will be a learning curve here, but your efforts will be rewarded.

Consume a cruciferous vegetable every day (cabbage, kale, broccoli rabe, cauliflower, arugula, Brussels sprouts, broccoli, broccoli sprouts, watercress, collard greens, bok choy or turnips). These vegetables contain high amounts of glucosinolate, a compound that sets them apart from other vegetables. Cruciferous vegetables help the liver to remove toxins that can block immune function. An added bonus is their ability to stimulate the production of enzymes that neutralize carcinogens, making them an important ally in cancer prevention. Read Appendix A. More about Cruciferous Vegetables on page 113 for an easy reference to this.

Protein is essential for immune support. Consume adequate protein. Excess protein does not confer any extra benefit and can be detrimental. To calculate your protein requirement for one day, multiply your weight in pounds by 0.36. If you are overweight, use your healthy weight for the calculation. Athletes will need slightly more, at least 0.54 grams per pound.

Eat dark leafy greens every day either in a large salad or lightly cooked. This will help fix many of your nutrient and fiber deficiencies. Experiment with dandelion, watercress and nettles. These are super-greens. Don't throw away the broccoli leaves. They are full of nutrients.

Caution:

If you are on a low-oxalate diet for health reasons, be aware that some green leafy vegetables are high in oxalates.

Twice a week, add a heaping teaspoon of ground flaxseed to a cup of water and drink it or to a bowl of steel-cut oatmeal for breakfast. Keep pre-ground flax in the freezer to prevent the fat from oxidizing, which causes it to become rancid.

Enjoy two or more daily cups of caffeine-free herbal tea, such as tulsi, turmeric ginger, or an immune blend. Or choose a blend that addresses your needs. You can find many herbal brands with names such as Throat Coat, Nighty Night and Breathe Easy. Green tea is also an excellent choice.

Eat meals and snacks at regular intervals. Skipping meals and then eating too much at the next meal will stress your ability to regulate your blood sugar.

Vary your sources of fats and oils. Use a combination of olive oil, coconut oil, avocado oil, pastured butter or ghee. Sesame oil can be added as a seasoning before serving as well. Flax oil is best used for salad dressing and other non-heated preparations.

Consume a fermented food every day. See page 41 for more on this.

Choose locally grown and organic foods, whenever possible.

Do not consume any foods that do not agree with you.

Do not snack frequently. Allow at least a three-hour interval between eating to support a healthy metabolism.

Use generous amounts of fresh and dried herbs.

Products I Love

- ♥ Bragg Organic Sprinkle. If you are new to exploring herbs and spices, I highly recommend this as a great seasoning blend to start with. It goes well with almost everything and offers a flavor that isn't overpowering.
- ♥ Penzeys Turkish Seasoning. If you enjoy a blast of flavor, this is great for marinades.
- ♥ Fourth & Heart ghee.
- ♥ *The Flavor Bible* by Karen Page and Andrew Dornenburg guides you as to what foods and seasonings complement each other.

Breakfast Ideas

○ Eat a raw vegetable with breakfast. When prepping dinner vegetables, fill a small container with uncooked vegetable pieces so it will be ready for the morning. If you are going to be physically active in the morning, it's okay to have fruit. The activity will metabolize the fruit, so it won't spike your blood sugar. Berries are low in sugar making them a good choice for everyone. If you can't do a raw vegetable yet, add a leftover, cooked vegetable. Plan ahead, make extra broccoli to add to an omelet.

○ Serve eggs sprinkled with nutritional yeast with leftover sliced yams in place of bread.

○ Top oatmeal with raw nuts or seeds, coconut oil and cinnamon.

○ Make extra soup so you will have leftovers. Lentil, vegetable and chicken soup make for a hearty cold-weather morning start.

○ Add sardines to a salad.

○ Spread almond butter on millet toast.

○ Prepare scrambled tofu.[19]

○ Spread bean dip on rice crackers or use as a vegetable dip.

○ Add quinoa to a bowl with berries and yogurt.

○ Top pancakes with berries.

○ Flavor plain yogurt with a sweetener and two drops of lemon essential oil. Top it with berries and hemp seeds.

○ Use unsweetened non-dairy milk to make a smoothie and add whey, pea, rice or hemp protein powder.

○ Add herbs, fresh or dried, as a topping for eggs, in tofu scrambles, on sardines or leftover soups.

---

19   Check out recipes at The Minimalist Baker (marieruggles.com/tofuscramble).

Consider adding a food high in vitamin C to boost your immunity right from the start of the day:

- ⮞ Sliced peppers (varied colors)
- ⮞ Mini peppers[20]
- ⮞ Tangerine
- ⮞ Cherry tomatoes (varied colors)
- ⮞ Blueberries mixed with raspberries

Lunch and Dinner Ideas

- ○ Plan ahead so you have ingredients on hand.
- ○ Have a large salad on most days. For added benefits and flavor, throw in chopped herbs, like parsley, basil or cilantro. Refer to "Think Outside the Salad Bowl" on page 26 for other ideas.
- ○ At least half of your plate should be filled with vegetables. This can include a side salad or a serving of fruit.
- ○ Diversify your fruit and vegetable choices and include all color groups.
- ○ Have some bean meals (split pea soup, bean-vegetable salad, bean chili). You can double- or triple-soak dry or canned beans to reduce gastrointestinal symptoms.
- ○ Limit red meat to twice a week, and buy grass-fed or organic if possible. This is more costly, but you can balance the cost by eating red meat less often and having a four-ounce portion size, which is enough for the average person. Feast on less costly legume (bean or lentil) meals several times a week. This will also help prevent getting cancer.
- ○ Purchase small fish to avoid the mercury that accumulates in large fish.
- ○ Consume two four-ounce servings of a fatty fish (salmon, sardines, anchovies, halibut or herring) weekly or take a daily 500 mg omega-3 supplement.

---

20 Eat them like fruit; no cutting required.

Sweet Treats

○ Make homemade baked goods using healthier choices, such as whole grains (oatmeal), vegetables (pumpkin) and zero-sugar sweeteners combined with regular sweeteners to reduce the sugar content.

○ Try dark chocolate with at least 65% cocoa or look for healthy recipes using cocoa, such as low-sugar brownies.

You may also want to visit recipes from the food bloggers recommended earlier for further ideas.

If you find yourself struggling with cravings, the deep cell nourishment that comes from eating whole foods will supply the fuel your body truly needs. Once you are eating mostly whole foods, it may take some time to build up the nutrient reserves your body is hungering for. Don't let that stop you. All along the way your body will be thanking you.

According to Sayer Ji, author of *Regenerate: Unlocking Your Body's Radical Resilience Through the New Biology*, the chocolate industry has been linked to trafficking. To purchase ethical chocolate, look for the Rainforest Alliance certification. Or opt for USDA-certified organic products, as nonorganic chocolate can contain residues of glyphosate. Avoid West African-sourced cacao.

Color Your World

THERE IS AN EXHAUSTIVE BODY of research confirming the myriad benefits of eating colorful fruits and vegetables. Each different pigment (blue, purple, red, orange, green, yellow, black and white) in the produce family represents a different group of anti-inflammatory and other bioactive compounds. By consuming colorful whole foods throughout the day, your cells are bathed in a robust supply of these health-enhancing compounds. Research indicates that brightly-colored fruits and vegetables boost immunity better than most supplements.

Plants are also met with wellness challenges and respond by developing their own warrior compounds to help them withstand illness. When you consume plant foods, those warrior compounds go to work in your body to build resilience.

The plethora of bioactives in colorful foods have a profound impact on bolstering immune function. The command center for your immune system resides in your gut. That is where a fountain of defense compounds are generated. Compounds from plant pigments are metabolized in the gut to feed your immune soldiers. This provides your body with a reserve of militia to get the job done with efficiency.

In addition to the palette of colors in fruits and vegetables, there are other colorful plant-based foods to choose from to expand your diet. Include the full spectrum of colorful plant-based foods, such as spices, whole grains, nuts and legumes in your snacks and meals to feed your body with the greatest possible variety of cell nutrients.

Other Plant Foods Providing Bioactives in a Variety of Colors

- ᴥ Cocoa: brown
- ᴥ Coffee and tea: brown, white, green, yellow, pink
- ᴥ Beans, dried peas, lentils: black, red, white, tan, pink, green, yellow
- ᴥ Nuts and seeds: tan, white, green (Think pistachios!)
- ᴥ Olives: black, green, purple
- ᴥ Quinoa: red, yellow, black, white
- ᴥ Rice: black, purple, tan, red, white

. . . .

☝ As you approach the grocery store checkout, do a review of the color status of your cart. Ultimately, I would love to see you indulge your cells with a bath of color-based bioactives every day, but let's start with where you are today. Will your current food haul allow you to consume at least three different colors today or tomorrow? If you currently only eat one color on a typical day, aim for two. Then gradually increase, doing whatever is manageable for you. My goal is for you to eat five different colors daily.

Juice Bathing

THIS IS HUGE. IT'S OKAY if juicing doesn't fit into your life. It's another project. I get it. That is exactly why I developed this technique. I find juicing to be incredibly beneficial, but a lot of work. So, I figured out how to minimize the chore while literally bathing my cells with hydration, nutrients and other bioactives for two days straight with a minimum of effort—**juice bathing!**

In this technique, you simply prepare juice once a week. Make enough for two days or more for sharing. Store extra in a large, covered jar. One day's serving would fill a large glass. Now here's the trick. Take one sip every (waking) hour over two days. This will immerse your cells in a continuous bath of antioxidants, anti-inflammatories and bioactives, a hydrating cocktail of delicious whole-body nourishment while spreading out the impact of any sugar in the fruits and vegetables you use.

Here are a few ideas on how to get started.

Many people buy juicers and never use them. So, it's easy to find a used, affordable juicer online. I purchased Breville's the Juice Fountain Cold XL on sale for $329. Why that one? My sister recommended it because it's easy to clean. I had another juicer that got little use because it was a nightmare to clean. I did some research, checked the ratings, and have been very happy with it. Since I only use it once a week for juice bathing, it's doable and the dividends are worth it. I feel healthier as I'm sipping the juice I make. So much so, that it's hard to not gulp down the entire glass of goodness at one time. But I restrain myself, knowing my cells are benefiting tremendously from the continuous supply of hourly sipping.

Once a week you can provide two days of cell love with a minimum amount of work. The added benefit of sipping instead of gulping it down is avoiding a sugar overload. Sweet vegetables, such as carrots, make a delicious juice, but the final beverage can be quite high in sugar. Juicing concentrates the sugars as it's removing the pulp. I love juicing carrots, but combine them with generous amounts of low-sugar vegetables (celery, cucumber, fennel) to balance out the final product.

Most of my students make juice bathing a weekend habit. They make the juice on Saturday morning and sip it hourly (or at whatever times are convenient) through Sunday night.

Try to use mostly organic produce. Keep it simple by only using three ingredients per drink. Purchase a few ingredients, then see what's in your refrigerator. Do you have a vegetable in there that's going to go bad if you don't eat it soon? Throw it in.

. . . .

   👍 Start with small amounts of ginger or turmeric root as they can impart strong flavors. Use only small handfuls of parsley or any green leafy vegetable or it may taste too "green."

If you happen to transition into the habit of daily juicing, it is very important to vary what you use. Juices provide a concentrated source of thousands of compounds. It is therefore best to add variety if you are juicing daily to avoid too much of a good thing.

A typical winter blend I make is carrots, celery and apple. Ginger and garlic are added if I need to boost the immune power of my juice.

Here are some ingredients I use for juicing. Don't get too hung up on amounts. Just play with it and discover what works for you. For the basic recipe, use one item for the base liquid, such as celery, carrots or cucumbers. Then, add in two other items.

Ingredient Options for Juicing

Vegetables

- Broccoli sprouts
- Cabbage (white or purple)
- Carrots
- Celery
- Cilantro
- Cucumber
- Fennel
- Greens (kale, etc.)
- Microgreens
- Parsley
- Romaine lettuce
- Tomato

Fruits

- Apple
- Berries
- Kiwi
- Lemon
- Lime
- Orange
- Pineapple
- Watermelon

Spices

- Garlic
- Ginger
- Turmeric

Think Outside the Salad Bowl

ANOTHER GREAT WAY TO INCLUDE more colorful whole foods in your diet is to have a large salad every day. Salad doesn't have to be the same all the time. Here are some ideas to mix it up with flavor and variety.

Start with Mixed Greens

- For a fast and easy salad use pre-washed blends.
- Use lettuce mixes with some dark greens, plus a variety of colors.
- Enhance pre-mixed blends by adding arugula, baby kale, endive or radicchio.
- Kale makes a great salad base by itself, but needs a little extra attention. Add olive oil and gently massage the leaves for fifteen seconds to allow them to soften. Let it sit for

thirty minutes before adding other ingredients. To lighten it up, add shredded white cabbage. Baby kale is more tender and doesn't need massaging.

○ Experiment with lettuce-free salads by chopping tomatoes, cucumbers, purple onion and basil. This is great as a side salad or a topping for a pesto-pasta meal.

○ Herbs, such as basil, parsley, mint and cilantro, liven up a salad while seriously upping the nutrient content.

Liven Up Your Salad with These Toppings

Vegetables

- Artichokes, marinated
- Beets
- Broccoli "slaw"
- Broccoli florets
- Broccoli sprouts
- Brussels sprouts, shredded
- Carrot, shredded
- Cauliflower crumbles
- Celery
- Cress
- Cucumber
- Fresh or dried herbs, like parsley, basil or cilantro
- Fresh peas
- Jicama
- Microgreens
- Olives
- Pea tendrils
- Peppers, use a variety of colors
- Purple cabbage, shredded
- Red onion
- Scallions
- Tomato, fresh or sun-dried

Proteins

- Almonds
- Black beans
- Black-eyed peas
- Chickpeas
- Grilled fish
- Kidney beans
- Pecans
- Pignolia nuts
- Pistachios
- Pumpkin seeds (pepitas)
- Sardines

- Sesame seeds (tan and black)
- Sunflower seeds
- Tofu
- Walnuts

Fruits

- Apple
- Berries
- Dried apricots
- Dried cranberries
- Grapes
- Kiwi
- Mango
- Orange
- Pear
- Raisins

According to Andrew Weil, MD, some mushrooms, including the common supermarket "button" variety, contain toxins. He recommends choosing from the wide variety (shiitake, cordyceps, enoki, maitake) of culinary mushrooms instead. Raw mushrooms are not on my list because they have very tough cell walls that are indigestible. Cooking the mushrooms will neutralize any toxins and release their nutrients.

Make your own salad dressing with extra virgin olive oil. This will help you avoid the overly processed oils used in commercial salad dressings. Bring your dressing to restaurants or request olive oil and vinegar, as they typically use salad dressings made with commercial (damaged) oils, such as corn, sunflower and canola.

Salad Combinations to Try

Mix any of these into an ordinary lettuce salad to bring the color and flavor up a notch:

- Cucumber, red onion, basil.
- Walnuts, dried cranberries,[21] apples, celery. (Add a touch of real maple syrup to the dressing.)
- Canned pears and pecans. (Drain syrup off pears.)
- Oranges, slivered almonds, dried cranberries. (Use orange juice in place of vinegar.)

---

21 Go light on dried fruit (raisins, cranberries) since this is a concentrated sugar.

- Scallions, sesame seeds, ginger dressing.
- Tomato, basil, olives, marinated artichoke.
- Avocado, cherry tomatoes and cilantro. (Add lime juice to the dressing.)
- Sliced beets, goat cheese, pecans.
- Figs, shredded Brussels sprouts, cress.
- Red onion, sun-dried tomato, basil.
- Chickpeas, red and yellow pepper, mango, cilantro.
- Apple, pear, walnuts, raisins.[22] (Add a little real maple syrup to the dressing.)
- Red and orange peppers, pignolia nuts. (Top with grated parmesan or Locatelli cheese.)

With any new food, start with a small amount and advance your intake slowly. Since you are biologically unique, your system is going to love some new foods and not others. This is good guidance for any new item you are planning to add. The benefits you receive from any healthy food will only be as good as your body's ability to digest and absorb it. If you have any signs of gastrointestinal problems, it is very important to resolve that as part of your overall wellness plan.

Foods That Can Hinder Immune Function

BIOLOGICALLY, WE ARE ALL DIFFERENT. What works for me, may not work for you. Consuming foods that don't agree with your physiology will weaken your immune system and derail your health in general. The most common offending foods are dairy and gluten (wheat and certain grains). Corn, eggs and soy can also be problematic for some people.

Food sensitivities can increase inflammation and derail stomach function. Your gastrointestinal tract is the control center of your immune response. Any food you have a sensitivity to can have a profound effect on your defense system and your overall health.

---

22   See footnote 21.

You may even have food sensitivities that you are unaware of, that is until you eliminate the offenders and feel noticeably better. Work with a nutrition-minded practitioner to be tested for your specific sensitivities. (Consult the organizations in "Medical Resources" on page 122 if you need to find a suitable practitioner.) Don't be afraid to learn about your food sensitivities. The market for alternative products has become so expansive, you may never look back at the dairy and gluten products you once loved and thought you couldn't live without. In the meantime, consider eliminating dairy or gluten if you have signs of a weak immune system.

I have witnessed drastic immune-health turnarounds simply by decreasing cow's milk and milk-containing products, such as processed cheese. Milk causes excess mucus in many people and drinking cow's milk is not good for most people. Small amounts of real (not processed) cheese, kefir and yogurt are okay, but regularly drinking cow's milk and eating a lot of factory-produced cheese is unhealthy for most people, whether they are lactose-sensitive or not. It creates an acidic environment and can increase inflammation, which plays a significant role in most diseases. Again, because there are so many different non-dairy milk alternatives, you may be surprised by what you taste and like. This change may not be as hard as you think.

The same is true for gluten, which is found in wheat and many other foods. This is especially problematic for anyone with an auto-immune condition. It is currently the consensus among nutritionists that gluten-containing products are detrimental to most people. It's challenging to make these changes, so I recommend starting with one at a time.

Here's why it's important. Anything that adversely impacts your health will pull energy reserves away from your immune system, which you need to combat viruses, inflammation and other adverse physiological reactions. It's important to avoid other foods as well that may be stressing or blocking the activity of your immune system, such as excess sugar, alcohol, foods with high pesticide levels, and fish with high mercury levels. Small fish don't live long enough to accumulate mercury, whereas large fish, such as tuna and swordfish, tend to be very high in mercury.

For additional guidance on making safer seafood choices, get the "Mercury in Fish" wallet card from the National Resources Defense Council at marieruggles.com/mercury.

The Environmental Working Group updates its two shoppers' guides annually. The first is The Dirty Dozen, which list the twelve foods with the highest pesticide levels (marieruggles.com/dirtydozen). The second guide is The Clean 15 and lists the fifteen foods with the lowest pesticide levels (marieruggles.com/clean15). Both are great resources to have.

Numerous studies have shown that sugar and refined carbohydrates derail immune function and damage the metabolism. Eating high-carbohydrate meals and snacks has a similar effect since white bread, pasta and rice are converted into sugar in the bloodstream. These high glycemic foods can lead to insulin resistance, a condition that leads to excess blood sugar because it has difficulty getting into the cell where it is needed for energy.

According to John Bagnulo, MPH, PhD, nutritionist, farmer and assistant professor:

> There's no faster way to suppress your immune system than to be insulin resistant. Excess insulin production, and the resistance associated with it, has repeatedly shown to predispose individuals for the highest risk for infections and severity of complications. Clearly, working toward a lower carbohydrate density diet, less sugar and lower glycemic foods is the path that offers the greatest returns to the immune system.

Sugar has been shown to diminish the ability of white blood cells to engulf and delete unwanted compounds. This effect occurs within less than thirty minutes after consuming the sugar and lasts for over five hours. Other refined carbohydrates include pizza dough, wraps, cookies, candy, juice, white flour, pastry, bagels, chips and most breakfast cereals.

Understanding Sugar on the Label

One teaspoon of sugar has four grams of sugar. So, if the label says "12 g sugar per serving," that equals three teaspoons of sugar. (12 g ÷ 4 = 3 tsp)

Sugar Alternatives

FORTUNATELY, THERE ARE VERY GOOD, natural sugar-free sweetener substitutes. Most of my students find these sweeteners work best when used in combination with each other or with natural sugar.

Experiment with a small amount the first time you try a new sweetener. Your preference for a sweet flavor is partly determined by your genetic makeup. What tastes pleasantly sweet to one person may taste awful to another. Whenever possible, sample a friend's sweetener before purchasing an entire container. Some people with digestive issues may find that a product causes gas and bloating. The natural sweetener stevia is intensely sweet and may send the wrong signals to your cells. If you use it, combine stevia with one of the more subtle sweeteners, such as monk fruit or erythritol, or use a pre-mixed blend.

Products I Love

- ♥ So Nourished Monk Fruit Erythritol Blend
- ♥ Lakanto Monk Fruit Sweetener (Golden) with erythritol
- ♥ Dragon Herbs Sweetfruit Drops
- ♥ NOW Real Food Organic Monk Fruit Liquid
- ♥ Whole Earth Sweetener Co Stevia Leaf and Monk Fruit

For natural sugars, small amounts of these are flavorful choices, but you'll want to be careful because they do have fructose and calories, and can increase blood sugar:

- Raw honey[23]
- Maple syrup or powder
- Longan (whole dried fruit)
- Molasses

Product I Love

♥ Coombs Family Farms Pure Organic Maple Sugar

Typically when I'm baking, I use a small amount of brown sugar plus Lakanto monk fruit sweetener. For other preparations, I often combine liquid monk fruit extract with Lakanto. If more flavor is needed, a small amount of maple syrup or maple granules does the trick.

Longan adds a wonderful flavor along with its subtle sweetness. It has a rich history among the Chinese who used it to build energy, calm the mind, add luster to the skin, promote deep refreshing sleep, increase circulation, and warm your hands and feet.

I like to add it to the water I boil for tea or put it into a pot of oatmeal while it's cooking. The longan can then be consumed along with the oatmeal.

Note on Coconut Products

Despite widespread recommendations, I am not a big fan of consuming large amounts of coconut products if you do not live in a tropical climate. The coconut's nutrient profile may be more suitable in large amounts only for people who live in regions where the trees thrive.

The water, flesh and milk are good to include in your diet in moderate amounts. The fat has a nice flavor and doesn't degrade with high flame cooking due to its high

---

23 Whenever possible, purchase raw honey from a local supplier. Many people with seasonal allergies find local honey helps decrease their symptoms.

smoke point. It's a tasty option for using along with vegetables and ginger, curry, cumin and other flavorful spices. It's okay to use it up to twice a day.

Be careful of recommendations to consume large amounts of trending foods. That's all they usually are—a trend. Unless, of course, we are talking about cruciferous vegetables!

A Note on Anti-Inflammatory Foods

THESE ARE A SPECIAL GROUP of foods that can help your body manage inflammation levels. A bit of inflammation is sometimes helpful, such as when you injure your knee and it gets red and swollen. This is a visible sign of the body's healthy repair response, and it involves short-term inflammation.

Long-term full-body inflammation is another story. Excess inflammation (also known as "chronic inflammation") may cause serious damage and can create a pathway for encouraging infections to be more aggressive. Excess weight is a common cause of chronic inflammation.

Many of us have chronic, low-level inflammation that we don't even feel. It's still doing damage though, even when it's not noticed.

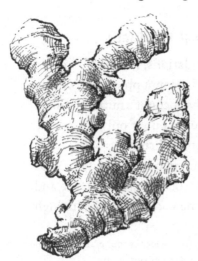

That's why it is important to include anti-inflammatory foods every day in your meals and snacks.

Following the recommendations in the "Whole Foods Quick Start Guide" will provide anti-inflammatory foods at every snack and meal. However, the foods highlighted on the next page provide extra support for reducing inflammation. Choosing an assortment of colored foods is a great starting place.

- 🌿 Avocados
- 🌿 Beans
- 🌿 Berries
- 🌿 Cocoa
- 🌿 Cruciferous vegetables
- 🌿 Ginger
- 🌿 Leafy greens

- 🌿 Mushrooms
- 🌿 Nuts
- 🌿 Sardines
- 🌿 Seeds
- 🌿 Sweet potatoes
- 🌿 Turmeric
- 🌿 Wild salmon

Excess meat (especially factory-farmed meat), excess sugar, artificial sweeteners, excess dairy, and processed foods create inflammation in your body.

Concerns about Cooking and Storage Containers

PLASTICS AND ALUMINUM LEACH HARMFUL compounds into your bloodstream that can build up over time and cause inflammation, as well as disrupt immune activity. These are at the root of many adverse health conditions. Use glass and stainless steel for food storage.

All plastics, including those labeled as BPA free, leach chemicals directly into your food. *Never* heat foods in any type of plastic.

Avoid aluminum cooking pans and foil trays. Did you ever notice tomato sauce erodes aluminum foil? Those eroded particles wind up in your sauce—and then in your brain. Use stainless steel, cast iron or glass cookware.

You may even consider bringing your own safe doggy bag or takeout container to restaurants. Otherwise, immediately transfer the food to a safe container as soon as you get home.

. . . .

👍 As an added reward for following my suggestions to nourish your immune system, your brain will benefit by improving your mood, your memory and your overall cognitive function.

CHAPTER 3. SUPERFOODS THAT OPTIMIZE GUT HEALTH & IMMUNE FUNCTION

In this chapter, you will learn about foods and beverages that reinforce your immune system by pushing your body to work at a higher level. This will enable you to further build your kitchen pharmacy and expand your home inventory of natural wellness options. All the suggestions in Chapters 2 through 5 work together to collectively prime your immune system and derail viral activity in your body. For your kitchen pharmacy, I have included mostly items that are easily accessible at your grocery stores or from online retailers like those listed in "Online Health Food Stores" on page 121.

Superfoods contain nutrients and bioactives that build resilience and strengthen baseline immune function when used regularly. Some really shine for specific short-term missions, such as when you have been near a sick person or feel like you have a cold or some other virus coming on. These powerful superfood compounds join forces with your biological warriors (white blood cells) to bolster immune activity. These rapid response options are also listed in Chapter 6, so you can easily identify them while consulting the action plan steps.

Remember you are the owner of an extraordinarily complex and infinitely wise immune system. It knows exactly what to do, but sometimes needs reinforcements to work at maximum efficiency. Your kitchen is a great place to start looking for those reinforcements.

According to one of the researchers in a recent food-as-medicine study:[24]

> Nature has been of the most exceptional help and source of inspiration for developing... antiviral compounds, affecting several steps of the viral life cycle.

Wow! All this "exceptional help" may be sitting in your pantry right now!

The bioactives in superfoods work in multiple ways. They may help your body produce more of its own antiviral soldiers. If a virus makes it past your first line of defense (barrier supports, such as mucus membranes), superfood bioactives may block the virus from entering your cells. Your cells are where viruses aim to set up home and replicate. That's something we want to stop dead in its tracks. Some superfoods fill in nutritional gaps left by a poor diet or depleted soil. Others contain compounds that regulate metabolic pathways affecting immune function.

In the next section, you will learn about what nature has to offer in the realm of foods that strengthen, cleanse, modulate and activate your immune system. What we take into our body and how we live can even affect how our genes function. This is food-as-medicine at its best!

To receive the greatest benefit, find a few superfoods and beverages you can incorporate regularly into your diet. Frequent consumption of their beneficial elements will saturate your cells in a pool of compounds that prime your immune system to be more resilient. By including probiotic foods regularly, along with a diverse selection of whole foods, you will also be strengthening the primary command station of your immune system, which lies in your gut.

---

24   Mohammadi Pour P, Fakhri S, Asgary S, Farzaei MH, Echeverría J. The Signaling Pathways, and Therapeutic Targets of Antiviral Agents: Focusing on the Antiviral Approaches and Clinical Perspectives of Anthocyanins in the Management of Viral Diseases. *Front Pharmacol.* 2019.

Most of the recommendations are for foods, with a few food-based supplements, such as elderberry syrup, nutritional yeast and grapefruit seed extract. This type of supplement naturally provides high concentrations of vitamins, minerals or bioactives. They are powerful and work well with your body because their biology is similar to what you are used to ingesting. They are not drugs and have an excellent safety record. There are other options, but this is what my work has primarily focused on.

I do have great respect for herbs; so I snuck in a few below and in Chapter 6. Seek out a clinical herbalist or naturopathic doctor for further guidance on expanding your wellness pantry with herbs. Consult "Resources" for other practitioners who utilize a broader range of nutraceuticals.

To keep the cost down, you can focus on your food choices. There's nothing more healing than homemade chicken soup prepared with love (and a few powerhouse spices). Refer to "Immunity on a Budget" on page 102 for more on this. Bon appétit!

Foods

Probiotics

Approximately 70% of your immune system resides in your gut, and probiotics (good bacteria) are at the heart of its activity. This area of immune artillery is referred to as your gut microbiota. A balanced presence of probiotics strongly influences immune system function, strengthens the stomach's protective barrier lining, and decreases the severity of respiratory infections. A review article in *Critical Care Medicine*[25] found that probiotics can help prevent the need for a ventilator in patients with pneumonia. This implies that one's microbiota may determine how severely you will react to a

---

25   Siempos II, Ntaidou TK, Falagas ME. Impact of the administration of probiotics on the incidence of ventilator-associated pneumonia: a meta-analysis of randomized controlled trials. *Crit Care Med.* 2010; 38(3):954-962.

viral infection. Simply put, establishing a balanced microbiota plays a vital role in preventing health complications.

According to John Bagnulo, MPH, PhD:

> The microbiota consists of microbe populations that either support or undermine our immune system. Eating ample vegetable fiber, providing some windows of time during the day without eating, and avoiding refined high-carbohydrate foods will often provide the kind of microbial balance that best supports the immune response and its effectiveness.

The goal is to continuously feed your microbiota to achieve a balanced, health-supporting mixture.

The first way to accomplish this is to diversify your food choices, eating a wide variety of colorful plant foods. In addition to fruits and vegetables, include a variety of beans, teas and spices in your quest to keep the microbiota healthy. Cruciferous vegetables play an important role in this since the fiber in vegetables and other plant foods feed your gut microbiota. They then manufacture additional compounds needed for protecting your health.

This process has such a profound influence on your overall health that Kathie Madonna Swift, co-founder of the Integrative and Functional Nutrition Academy and author of *The Swift Diet*, wrote:

> Since most of our immune system resides in the gastrointestinal tract, it is essential to nourish it with adequate fiber. Your microbiome will feast on fiber and, in turn, transform it into compounds that will support your health. The gut ultimately is your highway to health or pathway to pathology.

The second indispensable way to create a healthy probiotic balance is to include a daily serving of a prebiotic or a fermented food. Prebiotics are food for probiotics. They contain fibers that feed the probiotics already present in your gastrointestinal tract. The more prebiotic foods you eat, the healthier your gut will be. During the process of fermentation, foods develop their own supply of probiotics that are delivered directly to your gut upon consumption. Fermentation was traditionally used for food preservation.

Common fermented foods containing prebiotics and probiotics include:

Prebiotic Foods

- Almonds
- Asparagus
- Artichokes
- Bananas
- Beans
- Endive
- Garlic
- Greens
- Honey
- Jerusalem artichoke
- Jicama
- Kiwi
- Leeks
- Mushrooms
- Oats
- Onions

Fermented Foods

- Apple cider vinegar
- Cultured yogurt (dairy or non-dairy)
- Cured olives
- Fermented vegetables
- Kefir (dairy or coconut)
- Kimchi
- Miso
- Natto
- Raw cheese
- Sauerkraut[26]
- Tempeh

I recommend eating a fermented food every day. If you are new to fermented foods, the flavor can take a bit of getting used to. Start with a spoonful of fermented vegetables every morning. Even this small amount will have huge benefits. One of the milder blends, such as a carrot, ginger and cabbage, would be a good way to acclimate your taste buds. Try putting a spoonful on top of a salad.

---

26   The real type is often labeled "raw" and "unpasteurized."

Make sure the label says one of the following: "raw," "wild fermented," "unpasteurized" or "traditional method." These products will always be found in the refrigerated section of the supermarket. Beware! Some stores are putting shelf-stable, non-probiotic, non-fermented sauerkrauts onto the refrigerator shelves next to the truly fermented vegetable products. It is imperative to carefully scan the labels.

Miso paste is an easy and inexpensive way to get your daily dose of probiotics. Think of miso as salt and add it to anything you would add salt to instead of salt. It adds great flavor to bean dip, pesto and soups, especially bean soups. The easiest way to make sure you get a little every day is to add it to your salad dressing. Since it is a thick paste, miso needs to be thinned first with a small amount of water or whatever you're mixing it into. For hot foods, add it after the heat has been turned off and the food has cooled as the heat kills the probiotics present in any fermented food.

There is some preliminary evidence that hard Italian cheese may be a source of probiotics. A 2017 study reported the presence of small amounts of probiotics in Parmigiano-Reggiano cheese. These findings are only true for the Parmigiano-Reggiano from Italy with the Protected Designation of Origin certification, indicating the cheese had been made following a strict set of rules and only in a specified region.

A healthy probiotic balance can be upset by medication (especially antibiotics and oral contraceptives), excessive alcohol, processed foods and emotional distress.

. . . .

👍 An added benefit of working to build a healthy microbiota will be decreased inflammation. Chronic inflammation is a primary cause of disease.

> **Product I Love**
>
> ♥ South River Miso. This family-owned company makes miso according to the traditional Japanese farmhouse method. They offer delicious miso varieties including brown rice, dandelion leek, chickpea and azuki bean.

Elderberries

MY INITIAL EXPERIENCE WITH ELDERBERRIES was as a food in the form of syrup. I used it as a flavoring for plain yogurt, as pancake syrup, and in place of honey. These are simple ways to incorporate the firepower of this amazing antiviral berry into your families' winter menu.

Many herbalists and other practitioners think of elderberries as an herb. In addition to being widely available as a syrup (to be kept refrigerated), it is also available in a variety of other preparations, such as capsules, powder and gummies. All forms are good. It's simply a matter of personal preference. I love elderberries so much that my kitchen pharmacy is stocked with all forms.

So, what's all the well-earned buzz about these deep purple-black berries? They are rich in vitamin C and quercetin (more on this below) and contain a variety of vitamins and minerals, including zinc and magnesium. You will see vitamin C, zinc and magnesium are each on my essential immune nutrient list in Chapter 4. Elderberries reduce inflammation and contain potent antiviral compounds. They have been shown in clinical studies to combat infectious bronchitis and may help to prevent an infection from progressing to pneumonia.

There is an extensive body of research supporting the immune regulating properties of elderberries, and I consider them to be an essential component of my first line of defense for all things related to winter wellness. Think of elderberries as a daily shield of protection during times when viruses are going around.

It can be confusing to navigate the selection of products out there. My students have taught me there is no single form that's right for everyone. Many adults love the gummies. That's okay; the most important thing is to use a form that's going to be used as needed. If the candy-like taste of the gummies works for you, then that's fine. I love the formulation of some elderberry gummies that provide the added antiviral benefits of additional vitamin C and zinc in small amounts. The syrup is flavorful, but comes with a serving of sugar. Capsules are easy, and the powder can be used to enhance water. Using the powder to make tea is my favorite preparation because it provides a tasty way to bathe your cells in antiviral elderberry goodness all day long.

Each company has a different method for detailing the information related to the elderberry content and dosing of their product. Some products will include the term "standardized" on the label, but this level can change after the product has sat on a shelf. Instead of confusing you with these details, I'm going to recommend products from two companies I trust below. You can feel safe following their dosing recommendations. You can also double the dose if extra immune support is needed. During these times, your body may provide clues that you are coming down with something, such as an itchy throat, slight congestion or fatigue.

I recommend using elderberries every other day preventively when a virus is circulating in your community. Use them daily if you have a high level of exposure—like teachers during the winter or when you need to boost immune function when you have been near a sick person. Remember, the viral strategies in this book are all about getting ahead of the virus and not allowing it to gain a foothold in your body. It is for prevention, not treatment of illness.

Products I Love

- ♥ Gaia Herbs Immune Shine. This powder includes elderberries, mushrooms and ginger, making it a great immune-support blend. See the next page for my Immune Shine tea recipe.
- ♥ Gaia Herbs Black Elderberry (syrup or capsules)

- ♥ Gaia Herbs Black Elderberry Extra Strength Immune Support (gummies)
- ♥ Nature's Way Sambucus is an elderberry gummy that also contains zinc and vitamin C for extra immune support, which is a simple way to include other essential immune nutrients that are difficult to get enough of through diet alone.

Here is my favorite way to consume Immune Shine, a warm, comforting tea. It can also be mixed into a cup of ginger tea or blended with water and a scoop of vitamin C powder. Or you can empty the powder from a vitamin C capsule into the drink.

The best way to consume it is over several hours. This will provide your body with a continuous infusion of immunity-strengthening goodness. I like to put the tea into an insulated cup so it keeps warm for several hours at my desk.

Immune Shine Tea

1 cup warm water

1 teaspoon raw honey

1 teaspoon Immune Shine

1 teaspoon fresh lemon juice

Mushrooms

MUSHROOMS ARE THE EPITOME OF the food-as-medicine concept. They have been used for their medicinal properties for over 2,000 years. From a cooking perspective, they add an amazing culinary element to soups and stir-fries. Medicinally, they contain compounds that activate immune activity at many different levels—akin to one group of soldiers simultaneously fighting seven battles. Mushrooms are known for their wide array of bioactives, most notably their immune-enhancing polysaccharides. Note they are also included on the prebiotic list on page 41.

Beta-glucans are the specific polysaccharide responsible for boosting natural killer-cell activity and for activating the surveillance activity of warrior cells. The most studied mushrooms are turkey tail, maitake, shiitake and reishi.

Mushrooms are delicious, as well as good for you, and research shows they play an important role in modulating immune function. They also have anti-cancer properties, so mushrooms make a smart addition to any menu.

According to Donnie Yance, CN, MH, RH, clinical master herbalist, certified nutritionist and cancer specialist:

> Consumption of mushrooms and mushroom products in our daily diet provide profound health benefits, including the potential to significantly reduce cancer risk.

Aim to include mushrooms in your meals at least twice a week by cooking enough so you will have leftovers. During times of increased immune vulnerability, see if you can up it to three times a week. Alternatively, you can add a mushroom supplement to fortify your cells with a consistent supply of mushroom wisdom.

Mushrooms should be cooked to neutralize a toxin present in its raw state. If you are new to using mushrooms, start with any variety that's available at your local market. Grill or sauté them in butter, coconut or olive oil before incorporating them into a vegetable, pasta sauce or soup. Sauté them in the same pan you will be using for the remainder of the meal, so all the flavor is kept in one pot. Bonus... one less pot to clean!

Mushrooms are also available as teas, powders and liquid extracts.

Products I Love

- ♥ Natura Health Products Mushroom Synergy
- ♥ Host Defense MyCommunity (extract or capsules)

Curcumin

CURCUMIN IS THE DEEP-YELLOW BIOACTIVE compound responsible for all the well-earned excitement surrounding turmeric. In food-as-medicine terms, **turmeric** is the culinary spice, while **curcumin** is the medicine present inside the spice. Turmeric is a component of curry spice blends used in Indian foods. You may already be consuming it in mustard since turmeric is what gives it the yellow color.

Curcumin is the most widely studied plant compound with almost 15,000 studies listed on PubMed at the time of this writing.

Some researchers attribute the low incidence of cancer in India to their daily use of turmeric in cooking. Curcumin may be the most potent substance in your kitchen pharmacy. It has been shown in numerous clinical trials to be a powerful anti-inflammatory that controls the genes that suppress the spread of cancer. It has also been used to treat Alzheimer's, heart disease, diabetes and arthritis.

The anti-inflammatory activity of curcumin is so important because inflammation plays a significant role in most diseases. You can also have inflammation without even being aware of it, known as chronic low-grade inflammation. Viral infections are sometimes driven deeper into a person who has chronic inflammation. It can exacerbate infections and impede the body's ability to wage a strong defense against them. Chronic inflammation is comparable to spreading glue on your internal immunity battlefield!

Given the remarkable safety record for curcumin and its manifold health-protective attributes, I recommend daily use of turmeric, consumption of curry powder, or supplemental turmeric. The challenge with fully benefiting from turmeric is related to its poor absorption. Many nutritionists like to say you are what you eat, absorb and assimilate. The absorption of curcumin can be enhanced by including black pepper and a fat or oil in the same meal.

Be cautious when purchasing turmeric, though. Sometimes, it is contaminated with lead, which is added for the purpose of making it more yellow.[27] Ask the company you purchase turmeric or curry powder from if it has been analyzed for heavy metals.

One of my favorite ways to get a daily dose is to add a teaspoon of turmeric powder to a bottle of salad dressing. My salad dressing always contains olive oil and pepper, so that takes care of the absorption issue. Most people benefit from eating a large daily salad with homemade dressing. If you don't make your own dressing, you can still benefit by adding the turmeric and pepper to your bottle (along with miso).

The second way to get a dose of well-absorbed curcumin is by making curries. Several companies offer curry pastes you can simply add to coconut milk along with vegetables and a protein for a quick one-pot meal.

Third, powdered curry spice can be cooked in two or three teaspoons of coconut oil or ghee and onions for a few minutes, and then tossed with a cooked vegetable. The spice can be used to flavor other dishes, such as pureed winter squash soup, by adding in other compatible ingredients, such as ginger, black pepper, garlic and coconut oil. The bioactives work as teammates, each conferring more protection than they would on their own. And you may find your dishes will be elevated to an entirely new level of yum!

The fourth option is to take a curcumin supplement that is in an absorbable form or combined with other health-enhancing ingredients, such as green tea, ginger, black pepper, quercetin and rosemary. Taking curcumin as a supplement is a case where science may improve on nature, possibly trumping the benefit of the naturally occurring curcumin medicine in the spice powder. Some comprehensive curcumin products, such as the first product listed below, are thought of by nutritionists as the equivalent of a daily multivitamin supplement, except more herbal in composition. They offer an investment in long-term wellness by protecting cell health at every

---

27 Forsyth JE, Nurunnahar S, Islam SS, et al. Turmeric means "yellow" in Bengali: Lead chromate pigments added to turmeric threaten public health across Bangladesh. *Environ Res.* 2019.

level including healthy cardiac and neurological support. The synergistic composition of these products serves to amplify the benefits of the other ingredients. Additionally, the enhanced absorption and convenience for those who are not accustomed to daily curry consumption can confer amazing, overall health benefits.

Products I Love

Curcumin Supplements

♥   Natura Health Products Botanical Treasures

♥   Life Extension Super Bio-Curcumin

Curry Powder

♥   Simply Organic Curry Powder

Colostrum

COLOSTRUM IS AN IMMUNE-ENHANCING COMPOUND produced in the milk of humans, cattle and other mammals. It's high in protein, antibodies and white blood cells, which protects newborns from infections.

These same compounds contribute to its strong immunity-enhancing properties when taken as a supplement. It has been found to be healing to the digestive tract and contains growth factors that make it popular as a muscle-building supplement. It also plays a role in balancing the gut microbiota, which we explored in Chapter 3, for its profound effect on boosting the immune system.

Cow colostrum is the most common source of the supplement form. When it is dried into a powder, most of the lactose is removed. This type of product is often referred to as "bovine colostrum" and is typically incorporated into smoothies.

I recommend taking colostrum as a daily supplement in the form of a beverage, preferably one that is combined with other ingredients that work synergistically to nourish, build immunity, support gastrointestinal health, and stimulate fat metabolism while enhancing lean muscle and overall body composition—all of which serve to strengthen your resilience!

> ## Product I Love
> ♥   Natura Health Products Beyond Whey
>   (protein powder)

Nutritional Yeast

IN THE PAST, I REGARDED these little flakes as "hippie food," but not anymore after taking a close look at the science. Nutritional yeast undergoes a heating and drying process that renders the yeast inactive while maintaining its nutritive properties. It contains a host of vitamins and minerals, plus fiber and protein.

What makes nutritional yeast unique? It contains two important ingredients: the extensively-researched beta-glucans and nucleotides.

Beta-glucans enhance immune function by activating white blood cells—your immune system's first line of defense. This proliferation of warrior white blood cells is quite substantial. Remember, these "killer" cells attack, engulf and digest pathogens.

Nucleotides are an essential supplement for optimizing immune function. In a *Journal of Nutrition* review of dietary nucleotides, the authors state:

> ...nucleotides are biological molecules integral to almost all biological processes in the body. They are essential in many situations, such as during times of increased demands on the immune system.

In our toxic environment, our immune systems are always in need of extra support.

One study found that cyclists, who typically experience a drop in immunity after intense training, experienced an increase in immune cells as a result of consuming a mere ¾ teaspoon of nutritional yeast before cycling. The remarkable finding here was that the level of immune cells was actually higher than when they started cycling.

This immune-enhancing effect has been shown in other research with athletes. Elite athletes often experience a drop in immune function following an event. A study with runners found that those taking nutritional yeast did not experience the immune drop following a marathon. Additionally, they experienced an improved state of vigor and mood. Please pass the yeast!

Many committed users claim nutritional yeast has a nutty or cheesy flavor. Others find it can be used to enhance the flavor of most dishes. Each brand has a unique flavor profile. Nutritional yeast offers a multitude of B vitamins, except for B12, which some companies add in. The brand I recommend is not fortified in any way.

It can be used to season pesto, bean dip, popcorn, tomato-based sauces, bean soups, vegetables or added as a salad topper. Keep a small jar of nutritional yeast in your kitchen pharmacy and experiment with its pleasant flavor. I recommend using a half-teaspoon daily to add a nutrient and immune boost to your food. During times of immune vulnerability, use a teaspoon up to three times daily or try my Yeast & Sea Blend below. Your cells will thank you!

Only use brands that test for lead contamination and contain no genetically modified ingredients.

Product I Love

♥ Foods Alive Nutritional Yeast

Yeast & Sea Blend

This is a combination of nutritional yeast plus another favorite product, seaweed-enhanced sea salt. It's a great way to combine nutritional yeast's vitamin-mineral-bioactive nourishment with the immune-supportive iodine from seaweed plus sixty other trace minerals found in real sea salt. Simply combine the two ingredients and use it in the same way you would use a salt-containing spice blend. The proportions can be modified to suit your taste.

Yeast & Sea Blend

2 tablespoons Nutritional Yeast flakes

½ teaspoon Selina Naturally Celtic Sea Salt Gourmet
Seaweed Seasoning

Combine and place into a used spice jar with a wide opening
to make it easy to sprinkle onto your food.

Soup and Bone Broth

THERE IS NOTHING MORE NOURISHING than a warm bowl of soup. In
addition to the bone-deep healing comfort they impart, soups are
a great foundation for incorporating several immune-supporting
ingredients, such as:

- Basil
- Cilantro
- Chives
- Dill
- Garlic
- Ginger
- Hot peppers
- Leafy greens
- Lemon juice
- Lime juice
- Miso
- Mushrooms
- Nutritional yeast
- Onions
- Oregano
- Parsley
- Rosemary
- Scallions
- Seaweed

Broth, made from either meat or fish bones, is the most nourishing foundation for soup. During the long simmering of the bones
required to make real bone broth, the marrow releases stem cells,
which are used by your body to manufacture white blood cells.
Bones also release calcium and magnesium, plus a bath of bioactives
including collagen and glucosamine, which will strengthen your
bones, cartilage, hair, nails and joints. The glutamine it releases can
help heal leaky gut, a common gastrointestinal condition.

According to Sayer Ji, founder of GreenMedInfo and author of *Regenerate*:

> ...functional foods like chicken soup can support our bodies in their endeavor to heal—promoting resolution of acute illness and setting the stage for reversal of chronic illness. Foods can send your genes the equivalent of healing "text messages," providing a map for what your body has always known how to do—heal.

In clinical trials, soup has been shown to relieve upper respiratory tract inflammation and thin mucus. A remarkable study in the *Chest Journal* found chicken soup may have therapeutic effects in people with pneumonia. The authors stated:

> ...chicken soup may contain a number of substances with beneficial medicinal activity. A mild anti-inflammatory effect could be one mechanism by which the soup could result in the mitigation of symptomatic upper respiratory tract infections.

If you avoid meat and fish, a broth can still be made with a mixed vegetable base, along with the addition of a few ingredients from the list above. It will still deliver deep nourishment. Or look up a recipe for hot and sour soup and include mushrooms, garlic and ginger with a dash of hot pepper, such as cayenne. This will give you a perfect blend of flavor, plus restorative plant compounds. If using tofu, go for the organic. All nonorganic tofu is genetically modified. Or if you prefer, make a light vegetable soup, especially if your stomach needs a rest. Let's face it, years ago, your grandma intuitively knew soup was the best medicine in her kitchen!

Making bone broth requires anywhere from two to twenty-four hours of simmering. The longer the bones simmer, the more goodness will be extracted. Only use the bones of organic, pastured poultry to avoid extracting any toxins that have lodged in the animal's bones. You can also opt to purchase pre-made bone broth. A real bone broth will thicken in the refrigerator, showing it was truly simmered long enough to release gelatin. Avoid purchasing broth in plastic containers that leach plasticizers into the broth.

> **Product I Love**
> ♥   Kettle & Fire Bone Broth (any variety)

👍 The authors of the study demonstrating chicken soup thins mucus, noted that the inhalation of the steamy soup before consumption may play a significant role in thinning mucus.

Foods with Flavonoids

FLAVONOIDS ARE BIOACTIVES PRESENT IN plant foods with structures similar to antiviral drugs. Plant foods that contain flavonoids have been found to improve immune resistance to viral infection.[28] This is all very preliminary, but it turns out the flavonoid-containing foods are excellent additions to your diet, as recommended elsewhere in this book. Further investigations are currently underway, but there's every reason to add more of these bioactive-rich foods to your meals.

Many foods contain flavonoids. Following are the ones mentioned in the research.

- Cabbage
- Chili pepper
- Citrus fruit
- Dill
- Fennel leaf
- Green teas
- Olives
- Onion
- Oregano
- Spinach
- Turmeric

---

28   Burkard M, Leischner C, Lauer UM, Busch C, Venturelli S, Frank J. Dietary Flavonoids and Modulation of Natural Killer Cells: Implications in Malignant and Viral Diseases. *J Nutr Biochem.* 2017 Aug; 46:1–12.

Grapefruit Seed Extract

STUDIES HAVE SHOWN GRAPEFRUIT SEED extract, which contains a high level of flavonoids, displays a range of antimicrobial action. It has been used for a variety of purposes related to infections since the 1960s. It is an ingredient in nutritional formulas for gastrointestinal health, including the treatment of candida. This food-based supplement is available in both liquid and capsule form.

Caution:

Grapefruit can affect the way your liver breaks down certain medications, so you should check with your pharmacist or doctor before consuming it if you are taking any prescriptions.

Products I Love

♥ NutriBiotic GSE Liquid Concentrate
♥ Pure Encapsulations Grapefruit Seed Extract

Foods with Quercetin

QUERCETIN IS A FLAVONOID WITH strong, antiviral properties. It is present in apples, red onions, black tea, berries (especially elder-berries), broccoli, dark chocolate, black currants, asparagus, green chili peppers, oregano, capers, cloves (as well as herbs and spices in general), tomatoes, leafy green vegetables, shallots and onions (especially red onions).

The PubMed database lists over 19,000 quercetin research studies. It has shown promise in many health conditions. A particularly interesting animal study looking at this flavonoid's effect on the flu suggested it prevents lung-tissue damage that can result from a viral infection. Additionally, quercetin reduces the incidence of secondary bacterial infections, the main cause of death in people with the flu.

Researchers suggest that quercetin's effectiveness is related to its ability to prevent viral infections or inhibit it if the infection does get into your cells.

Human studies have also been encouraging and researchers have noted that quercetin may be a promising treatment for the common cold. It has demonstrated the ability to inhibit a wide variety of viral infections, including the flu.

Quercetin supplements are most effective when combined with synergistic compounds, such as bromelain, to treat infections. Since this book is focused on prevention, not treatment, I recommend making quercetin-rich foods a daily component of your diet all year, so your body can build up reserves of this remarkable flavonoid.

. . . .

👍 Quercetin also helps manage seasonal allergies.

Foods with Anthocyanins

ANTHOCYANINS ALSO COME UNDER THE flavonoid category. Any super-food conversation would be incomplete without a special focus on anthocyanin-rich berries. You will find berries on the Top 5 list of any serious nutrition blogger. The anthocyanins are the pigments that give berries their rich color along with a host of health-supportive properties. These pigments include deep shades of purple, red and blue. Many other foods with intense pigments, such as spices and purple cabbage, also contain anthocyanins.

Berries have a lot of health benefits including preventing viruses from entering the cells.

I recommend the frequent consumption of fresh or frozen berries. Use them in smoothies, pancakes or just eat them as a nutritious snack. They can even be added to salads for a sweet and colorful touch.

Many people get their daily dose of anthocyanins by adding a teaspoon of a condensed berry powder or extract to water or mixed into anything that would be enhanced by a touch of sweetness. It can also be added to a "green" drink or smoothie. If you choose to use this type of product, make sure it's purely a mix of berries (preferably organic).

> **Product I Love**
>
> ♥ Natural Health Fruit Anthocyanins

Beets

BEETS HAVE EARNED A SECURE place in the superfood Hall of Fame. Why? They contain bioactives with many benefits, as well as play a role in augmenting immune function. They assist in nitric-oxide production, an important compound that has been shown to decrease virus replication. As if all that were not enough, beets also support lung function and brain health, due to their ability to boost circulating oxygen levels. And yes, beets also contain the infamous flavonoid bioactives.

Pre-cooked and peeled beets are convenient to keep on hand for salads. A few ounces of beet juice is another way to capture their benefits. Since the juice concentrates the naturally occurring sugar in beets, it's best to limit the amount to two ounces. More would be fine if you are headed out for some exercise.

Honey

HONEY HAS BEEN FOUND TO contain over 150 health-promoting bioactives. It can be useful for soothing throat irritation and is a wonderful addition to a warm cup of tea or even a cooled ice tea in the warmer months. Thick honey will need to be diluted in warm water before adding it to a cold liquid.

Pasteurizing honey kills the vital enzymes and good bacteria that make raw honey one of the world's universal superfoods, so raw honey is preferable.

Honey is a powerhouse that appears on the prebiotic list earlier in this chapter, but also contains probiotics. In addition, raw honey has powerful anti-inflammatory properties.

. . . .

👍 Many people find consuming locally-produced raw honey has the added benefit of helping to manage seasonal allergies due to the desensitizing effect of the tiny amount of local pollen present in the honey.

Ginger, Garlic and Oregano

HERBS HAVE BEEN USED AS natural remedies since ancient times. Most common kitchen herbs and spices have powerful antiviral effects against numerous viruses that cause infections in humans. Many have been the subject of clinical studies, including garlic, ginger, basil, sage, dill, thyme, peppermint, cinnamon, rosemary, clove and fennel—just to name a few. Turmeric, the subject of thousands of studies has already been discussed earlier in this chapter.

There is no question the use of herbs (fresh or dried) is a simple, inexpensive way to add flavor, variety and health enhancement to any meal, snack or dessert. Feel free to use all of them liberally. Consult *The Flavor Bible* for an excellent guide on which foods combine well with specific herbs and spices.

Make it a regular habit to use ginger and garlic in increased amounts anytime viruses are circulating in your community. Ginger has a long history of health and immune-supporting uses. It has traditionally played a major role in both Indian Ayurveda and traditional Chinese medicine.

Fresh ginger has an intense flavor. Younger roots, which are sometimes pink, have a more subtle flavor. Because it's so strong, when it comes to ginger's health-boosting properties, a little bit goes a long way.

An easy way to start using ginger and garlic is to mince both and cook them on medium heat in coconut oil with sliced onions. Use this as a base for stir-frying or mix into cooked vegetables. Some stores sell pre-chopped frozen ginger and garlic, which are wonderful time savers.

Historically, garlic has been revered for its antibiotic-like properties and, in research, has been shown to activate killer cells against viruses and cancer cells. Cooking with fresh garlic is best, but garlic powder also has benefits.

Here is a simple way to activate garlic's powerful compounds.

Chop & Hold Garlic

Chop, slice or press raw garlic.

Let it sit for 10 minutes before cooking with it. During the ten-minute holding period, the compounds that have been meshed together from chopping will work to create more powerful bioactives.

After the hold period, simmer sliced garlic in olive oil for three minutes.

Once it cools, store it in a glass jar in the refrigerator. The garlic and the garlic-infused oil will be ready to add to your vegetables or any dish. This will keep in your refrigerator for two weeks.

You can make this in a large quantity so it's ready to use anytime.

Product I Love

♥ Chef'n Garliczoom garlic chopper

An herb worth noting that has exceptional properties for immune support is oregano. In the distilled form, the oil is effective against respiratory viruses, such as the flu and other viruses that affect the lungs. It is available in pill form or as drops that can be mixed into water or honey. You will find oregano oil used in both immune support Phases II and III (covered in Chapter 6).

Products I Love

♥ Designs for Health Oil of Oregano
♥ Garden of Life *mykind* Organics Oil of Oregano Seasonal Drops

Beverages

Water

YOUR CELLS FUNCTION AT THEIR best when they are well-hydrated. Aim to drink water or herbal teas throughout the day. Start with two glasses upon waking and drink most of it before eating if possible.

Fluids also rinse pathogens from your throat down into your stomach acid where they may be inactivated. This confers additional benefits by disrupting the travel plans of a virus that is headed to your lungs. Some viruses sit in the throat for a few days before moving down to the lungs. Sipping warm tea throughout the day can provide extra support when needed.

To get an estimate of the minimum amount of water you should drink daily, divide your body weight by two. For example, if you weigh 150 pounds, aim for drinking 75 ounces of water daily (150 ÷ 2 = 75).

If you are home, fill a pitcher with your day's water requirement. This makes it easy to monitor your intake. If you will be out of the house, fill a large stainless steel bottle with water and aim to finish it before returning home.

I recommend increasing your intake of all fluids (water, tea and broths) when you have a greater need for upper respiratory tract support, such as an itchy throat or stuffy nose.

Tea

CONSUMING TEA HAS BEEN SHOWN to benefit the healthy functioning of several body systems, including the immune system. The antimicrobial effect of tea dates back to a 1906 military journal, which suggested that troops fill their water bottles with black tea to prevent typhoid fever.

More recently, research has shown that drinking green tea reduced the incidence of the flu in children and in nursing home residents who gargled with a green tea extract. This makes a lot of sense since immunologists often speak about viruses setting up house in the throat. Drinking the tea washes some of the pathogens down into the stomach acid where they may be neutralized and gargling exposes viruses in the throat to extended contact with the tea's anti-viral compounds.

Many teas have unique benefits, especially when combined into blends. Adding the zest of a lemon or orange to warm tea can help thin excess mucus.

Tulsi (also known as "holy basil") is one of my personal favorites. It has been revered in many cultures around the world for its medicinal properties. More recently, research has caught up with these traditional uses, affirming its effectiveness in a variety of wellness challenges. It has been shown to be calming and uplifting to the spirit, and to provide powerful support for the immune system. Why not enjoy a few cups of this every day—warm or chilled?

I recommend keeping a few of the teas listed below in your kitchen pharmacy to enjoy any time of the year and for when special needs arise.

- Chamomile
- Eucalyptus
- Ginger
- Green
- Pau D'Arco
- Peppermint
- Thyme[29]
- Tulsi

Check with any companies you purchase tea from to see what their tea bags are made out of. Some companies are using plastics for making their tea bags, which you'll want to avoid.

Here is one of my favorite ways to make an overnight tea with goji berries, the most nutrient-dense food ever analyzed.

Goji Berry Overnight Tea

1 tablespoon dried goji berries

8 ounces of water (room temperature is fine)

Place the berries and water into a mug. Let it sit overnight, and enjoy waking up to a deep berry-colored tea. Strain out the berries, and put them into another mug with water.

This can be repeated until the berries no longer create a berry-colored tea.

---

29   This is especially good when you want to clear extra fluid from the lungs.

> **Products I Love**
>
> **Tea blends with specific purposes**
> - ♥ Buddha Teas Organic Thyme Leaf
> - ♥ Choice Reishi Detox
> - ♥ Gaia Herbs Bronchial Wellness
> - ♥ Mighty Leaf Organic Detox Infusion
> - ♥ Organic India Tulsi Original
> - ♥ Organic India Tulsi Turmeric Ginger
> - ♥ Rishi Turmeric Ginger
> - ♥ Traditional Medicinals Breathe Easy
> - ♥ Traditional Medicinals Throat Coat (any variety)
> - ♥ Twinings Organic Peppermint

Coconut Water

COCONUT WATER IS NOT NECESSARILY a superfood per se, but I wanted to include it here because it can sometimes be beneficial. This will come in handy if you are under the weather and not drinking enough water or eating your usual healthy fare. Let's face it, we are not always up for slicing, dicing and cooking vegetables during these times.

Coconut water can serve two purposes here. One is hydration and the second is replacing some of the potassium you would normally get from vegetables. Keep coconut water on hand so this is easy to do. It has a high amount of naturally occurring sugar, so I recommend diluting it. Add 4 ounces of coconut water to 16 ounces of regular water and sip it over several hours. Repeat up to twice daily. Its sweet flavor will also encourage you to drink and remain sufficiently hydrated, which is especially important for upper respiratory support.

Caution:

Avoid coconut water if you have kidney failure.

CHAPTER 4. NUTRIENTS AND SUPPLEMENTS THAT OPTIMIZE IMMUNE FUNCTION

The nutrients and bioactives present in whole foods provide the foundation for priming your immune system. Yet even the most conscientious eater can fall short on key vitamins and minerals because the soil your food is grown on is most likely depleted. The most recent data from the United States Department of Agriculture (USDA) reveals many Americans are markedly deficient in key immune nutrients including vitamins A, C, D and magnesium.

Some of our nutrient deficiencies are also related to lifestyle. According to Diana Noland, MPH, RDN, IFMCP, LD:

> A majority of the United States population does not have the available nutrients to meet the essentials of a generally more stressed society.

In this chapter, you will learn how to stock your pantry with foods and supplements that will supply the nutrients you need to infuse your cells with immune-priming nutrients. These nutrients will provide the fuel for activation, renewal, detoxification and ultimately system optimization. Microbiologist and immunologist, Aristo Vojdani, PhD, has pointed out that your immune cells love nutrients; they even have receptors specifically for vitamins and minerals.

You can prime your immune system by ensuring your body has an adequate supply of the critical nutrients discussed below along with gradually replacing processed foods with whole foods.

You will learn about vitamin D, a key nutrient for supporting immune function. Then we will move onto a few other crucial vitamins and minerals that have repeatedly been shown in the research to strengthen immune function. Please remember all this builds upon a nourishing whole food, plant-focused foundation.

Some options below are great to work on every day or as much as possible. Other suggestions can be used when you need a short-term boost. (For example, increasing vitamin C when needed for extra immune support.) All these suggestions are for immune optimization and not intended for the treatment of any specific illness.

Vitamin D

VITAMIN D IS OFTEN REFERRED to as our universal guardian, but can require supplementation since it is nearly impossible to get adequate amounts from diet alone. It is also known as the "sun vitamin" because it can be synthesized in the skin from exposure to sunlight.

This nutrient directs gene behavior, with over 3,000 genes that rely on it for proper function. It's that important. Recent reports in the *International Journal of Molecular Science*[30] and *Reviews in Molecular Virology*[31] each identified vitamin D as a very important nutrient for supporting healthy immune function.

If you haven't taken a vitamin D supplement and it's the middle of winter, you are most likely deficient. The depletion of serum D levels, which reflects the amount of vitamin D in your blood, makes us more vulnerable to infections. Viruses are most common in winter, when vitamin D levels tend to be the lowest. The flu is a viral infection

---

30   Gruber-Bzura BM. Vitamin D and Influenza-Prevention or Therapy? *Int J Mol Sci.* 2018 Aug 16; 19(8):40–44.

31   Trymoori-Rad M, Shokri F, Salimi V, Marashi SM. The Interplay Between Vitamin D and Viral Infections. *Rev Med Virol.* 2019 March; 29(2):e2032.

that can affect the lungs. The authors of a 2015 study in the *Thorax* journal[32] stated:

> Vitamin D deficiency is common in people who develop ARDS (acute respiratory distress syndrome). This deficiency of vitamin D appears to contribute to the development of the condition, and approaches to correct vitamin D deficiency in patients at risk of ARDS should be developed.

Vitamin D boosts the production of white blood (fighter) cells. It also plays an important role in regulating inflammation, and numerous studies have demonstrated it's a critical nutrient for fueling robust immune activity.

A recent review[33] of twenty-five trials in the *British Medical Journal* demonstrated that individuals benefited greatly from vitamin D supplementation, especially those who started with very low levels.

Most people are not only deficient in vitamin D in winter, but all year round, especially if you have limited sun exposure, since your body makes vitamin D in response to sunlight. Even if you get a lot of sun, but most of your skin is covered or you are wearing sunblock, you may be deficient, and some people simply don't make enough vitamin D even with good exposure to sunlight. This includes people who are overweight or have darker skin tones.

It is well-documented that the darker the skin, the greater the probability of a vitamin D deficiency. Even in southern climates, 55% of African Americans and 22% of Caucasians are deficient. And even if you get a lot of direct skin exposure to the sun during the warmer months, your levels may plummet in the cooler months.

---

32   Dancer RC, Parekh D, Lax S, et al. Vitamin D deficiency contributes directly to the acute respiratory distress syndrome (ARDS). *Thorax*. 2015;70(7):617-624.

33   Martineau AR, Jolliffe DA, Hooper RL, et al. Vitamin D supplementation to prevent acute respiratory tract infections: systematic review and meta-analysis of individual participant data. *BMJ*. 2017;356:i6583. Published 2017 Feb 15. doi:10.1136/ bmj.i6583.

Some individuals have gene variants that cause an increased need for vitamin D.

Others who are at a higher risk for D deficiency include people:

- who have had bariatric surgery.
- with chronic inflammation.
- living at higher altitudes.
- on certain medications.
- who are pregnant or breastfeeding.
- who are over 60 years of age.

PubMed lists over 86,000 (!) vitamin D studies, with more being added all the time. The understanding regarding laboratory evaluation and safe dosing levels can change daily. What I'm presenting here is my current recommendation based on the evidence at the time of this writing. You can follow me on Facebook (Everyday Wellness Tools at marieruggles.com/facebook) to get evidence-based updates on dosing recommendations.

The Institute for Functional Medicine recommends aiming for 60-80 ng/mL of vitamin D in your lab evaluation. The specific name of the test you want to request is a "serum 25-hydroxy vitamin D." If you have had lab work requested by a nutrition-minded practitioner, they will guide you to the best level for your constitution and the starting amount of vitamin D needed to achieve that goal. If your practitioner is unable to guide you confidently, Grassroots Health, a major researcher into vitamin D, has a free online calculator you can easily use to determine the right dosage for your specific needs. You can learn more about it in "Vitamin D Dose Calculator" on page 123.

Conversely, if you spend a lot of time in the sun year-round, you may not need any supplementation at all; think of farmers in southern climates. Changing life circumstances (moving, losing weight, health problems, age, time of year) can all impact your needs.

For most deficient individuals, supplemental vitamin D is the only way to achieve an adequate level. Since individual vitamin D requirements vary, doses should be individualized. The most accurate way to determine how much to take is to have blood work done two to three times a year. Aim for the higher level if you have frequent lung infections; once at your yearly wellness checkup and then at four and eight months after that. By then, you will be due for your next yearly checkup.

After requesting a vitamin D level at your yearly wellness checkup, ask for two additional lab slips for checking it in the next four and eight months. If your initial vitamin D level is low and you are put onto a therapeutic dose, the next lab work will show if that dose is effectively raising your serum (blood) level. Many practitioners now utilize computerized systems where they can easily submit orders to your local lab for the additional tests during the year. There's no need to make an appointment just to get a lab slip. If your practitioner questions your request, inform them you are proactive in your healthcare and maintaining an adequate D level is a critical piece to this approach. If they have further questions, gently refer them to PubMed.

Whenever possible, I recommend getting your vitamin D from sunshine. Spending fifteen minutes, two to three days a week in the noon sun, with most of your body exposed (no sunblock), is a good way to increase your levels naturally unless you are elderly or dark-skinned, in which case you may require even more exposure. Individuals over age 65 may require up to three times more time in the sun to make an adequate supply of vitamin D. Since all of us are biologically different, this advice will vary, but it's a good starting place.

Vitamin D3 is the best form to take because it's more biologically compatible with human physiology. D3 is the form your body makes in response to sun exposure, and it is more effective for increasing the serum D level. However, not all D3 supplements are created equal. It is better if the vitamin D is combined with the vitamin K derivatives (K1 and K2) since they work as a team. Vitamin D increases the absorption of calcium. Vitamin K helps to usher the calcium into the bones, where it belongs. Without vitamin K, the calcium can wind up where it doesn't belong and wreak havoc in the arteries and joints.

How much vitamin D3 you take depends on many factors, including your current blood levels as well as your sun exposure, geographic location, and skin color. If you are unable to get a reading on your current level, the Institute for Functional Medicine recommends starting with a daily dosage of 5,000 IU and then to be tested as soon as possible.

It may take some experimentation to find the dosage that will keep you in the optimal range of 60 ng/mL. The dosage required to maintain this range may vary during the year. Deficient individuals are often given an initial high dose of 15,000 IU for the first three days to jumpstart the process of vitamin D repletion, and then 2,000 to 5,000 IU daily until retesting in three months. There is no one-size-fits-all when it comes to vitamin D dosing. Your personal, lifestyle, genetics and state of health determine the amount that is right for you.

Vitamin D is a fat-soluble vitamin and is better absorbed when taken with some fat or at your largest meal. One study found taking vitamin D with dinner increased blood levels of D 50% more than when it was taken with breakfast.

Why is all of this so important? Think of vitamin D as more of a hormone than a vitamin.

It helps manage inflammation and turns on genes that directly affect the functioning of your immune system.

If you have low immune function, it's even more important to be vigilant about monitoring your vitamin D level. Adequate nourishment at the cellular level will go a long way toward improving your health.

If you plan to use the sun to increase your D, limit your initial exposure to allow your body to rev up its ability to produce pigmentation that will give you some color while protecting you from overexposure to the sun. If you are light-skinned, limit your initial exposure to a few minutes.

. . . .

👍 A wonderful benefit of maintaining optimal D levels is it will reduce your risk of cancer, osteoporosis, high blood pressure, mood disorders and heart disease, just to name a few!

Caution:

Check with your healthcare provider before taking vitamin D supplements if you have a history of kidney stones, hypercalcemia, hyperparathyroidism, lymphoma (either Hodgkin's or non-Hodgkin's), granulomatous disease (sarcoidosis,) tuberculosis, kidney disease or liver disease. You'll also want to check with your practitioner if you are on medication or have any health condition where you need to be careful with your vitamin K intake. If you are on a blood thinner, remember that it is important to consume the same amount of vitamin K every day.

Products I Love

Vitamin D[34] with Vitamins K1 and K2
- ♥ Designs for Health Vitamin D Supreme with 5,000 IU of D

Vitamin D with Vitamin K2
- ♥ Seeking Health Vitamin D3 + K2 with 5,000 IU of D
- ♥ Ortho Molecular Products Liquid Vitamin D3 with K2 with 1,000 IU of D

Vitamin D Only
- ♥ Nature's Way Vitamin D3 with 2,000 IU of D
- ♥ Carlson Liquid Super Daily D3 drops with 1,000 IU of D

---

34 Some companies list vitamin D in micrograms (mcg). 25 mcg = 1,000 IU.

To save money, you can purchase vitamin D3 with only vitamin K2 and consume it with a food that's high in vitamin K1, such as broccoli, kale, mustard greens, swiss chard, collard greens or spinach.

Alternatively, you can save even more money by purchasing vitamin D3 without any vitamin K and consume it with a vitamin K1 food plus a serving of a K2 food. For example, eat a fermented vegetable, such as cabbage or natto (fermented soybeans), or aged cheese, such as authentic gouda, milner, cheddar, stilton, camembert, roquefort and cheese made from raw milk.

Vitamin C

HUMANS DO NOT INTERNALLY PRODUCE vitamin C, so we need to get it from outside sources because it is essential to our health. This is particularly true for immune optimization since vitamin C is needed for augmenting the production and function of your warrior white blood cells and other immune soldiers responsible for destroying pathogens. It plays a role in collagen production, which is an important element of barrier (skin) immunity.

Numerous studies over the past thirty years have demonstrated the antiviral influence of vitamin C and its role in reducing the risk and severity of infections. It also protects these warrior cells, extending their ability to kill off foreign invaders. Studies have shown vitamin C prevents an infection from getting more severe, such as preventing a cold or bronchitis from turning into pneumonia. It has also been shown in clinical trials to shorten the length of stay for patients in intensive care units.[35] The government is currently conducting clinical trials to gain more insight into this along with specific dosing recommendations.

Vitamin C may also prevent bacterial and viral infections. This is a nutrient you want circulating in your bloodstream all day, every day. It is also important to have an abundant supply during times when

---

35   Hemilä H, Chalker E. Vitamin C Can Shorten the Length of Stay in the ICU: A Meta-Analysis. *Nutrients*. 2019; 11(4):708. Published 2019 Mar 27.

enhanced immune support is needed to meet your body's increased demand for vitamin C. According to Russell M. Jaffe, MD, PhD, CCN, "Vitamin C is the most powerful antiviral agent that we know of."

Your body doesn't store vitamin C, so your supply is depleted every day, which means it needs to be replenished daily. It is depleted even more rapidly in people with health challenges, especially if they suffer from frequent infections.

Since vitamin C is a water-soluble nutrient, it is very safe to take several times daily. It's actually more beneficial to take it throughout the day than all at once. A reasonable daily dosage is 500-1,000 mg a day in divided doses. Most of us need to rely on a supplement to get a minimum of 500 mg daily.

The body uses more vitamin C during an infection. During times of increased need for immune support, I recommend 500 mg of vitamin C every two hours. See more on this in Chapter 6. Putting It All Together. Even if you eat an abundance of foods high in vitamin C, supplementation is the only way to reach the amount needed when you are aiming for this more therapeutic dose.

Supplemental vitamin C in doses above what can be achieved with food has been demonstrated to be valuable in improving the immune response to viral infection.[36] During times of increased immune-support needs, many practitioners recommend taking 1,000 mg/hour until diarrhea develops. Then the dose is decreased to the level that does not cause diarrhea. This is known as vitamin C "loading." They also use this technique to determine one's personal daily vitamin C needs, which can be up to 5,000 mg. This should be done under the care of a knowledgeable practitioner.

If you frequently need immune support, the proper dosage will be the one that helps you to feel healthy more consistently. Many practitioners and home-infusion companies offer intravenous (IV) vitamin C for supercharging immune activity during times of

---

36   Ran L, Zhao W, Wang J, Wang H, Zhao Ye, Tseng Y, Bu H. Extra Dose of Vitamin C Based on a Daily Supplementation Shortens the Common Cold: A Meta-Analysis of 9 Randomized Trials. *Biomed Res Int.* 2018 July 5; e1837634.

increased need. If IV vitamin C is not accessible (or affordable), they may substitute the liposomal form, which is less costly than IV, but still much more than the other choices recommended below.

Food is a great starting point for working toward your daily vitamin C goal because it comes packaged with a team of other anti-inflammatory compounds and bioactives meant to work together in your body. Because of the rich, synergistic combination of compounds present along with vitamin C in food sources, include a food from the list below every day to further enhance your vitamin C program and your health. Remember to "color your world" by choosing C-rich foods from several different color categories.

I enjoy starting my day with sliced peppers. It's easy on prep time and can be prepared the night before. When purchasing colored peppers, I also get all the benefits from the variety of bioactives present in each different pigment. Sometimes I even eat mini peppers like a fruit—just rinse and nosh. (Warning: You will get stares if you do this in public.) Another option I frequently enjoy is ending my lunch with a tangerine. It's simple and easy.

Try to eat some of the suggested options below in the raw form, since vitamin C is easily depleted during cooking. Simply eat more plant-focused meals and snacks and include a serving of at least one of these foods every day. To keep it simple, make a salad including two of the high-C options below, such as chopped parsley and peppers. Prep enough of these for a few days to save on time.

Food sources of vitamin C include:

- Citrus fruit and juice. Add lemon and lime juice to salad dressings and entrées for enhanced flavor (not to mention their cancer-preventive compounds).
- Peppers (all colors). Top grilled fish with chopped tomato, onion and peppers.
- Kiwi. Have as a pre-exercise snack or arrange on the side of a dinner plate to dress up the meal.
- Broccoli. Dip raw broccoli in hummus.

- ⊷ Parsley. Add a generous portion of chopped parsley to salads for an intense infusion of nourishment.
- ⊷ Snow peas. Pack these for a sweet, crunchy mid-afternoon snack.
- ⊷ Kale. Mix thinly-sliced kale into a salad; allow to stand for fifteen minutes to soften.
- ⊷ Acerola cherries. Plant a tree if you live in a warm climate.
- ⊷ Brussels sprouts. Slice thin and add to salads.
- ⊷ Tomatoes. Chop with basil and use as a topping for pasta with pesto.
- ⊷ Strawberries. Add to a spinach or kale salad.
- ⊷ Black currants (raw). Add to a fruit salad.
- ⊷ Cantaloupe. Slice and serve as an after-dinner treat.
- ⊷ Cauliflower. Roast and serve as an appetizer or side dish.
- ⊷ Cabbage. Add shredded cabbage to a salad.
- ⊷ Guava. Add a few chunks to a smoothie.
- ⊷ Potato, baked. Provides a small amount of C, but is a great option for those who are at the beginning of their vegetable journey.

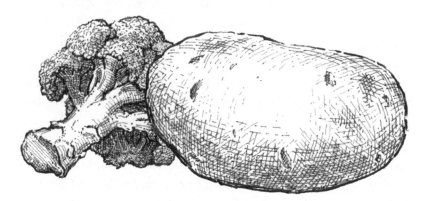

Oh, yeah! Can we get over our fear of potatoes? Check out my favorite nutrition and cancer blogger, Donnie Yance at marieruggles.com/yancepotatoes to see what he has to say about the humble potato.

By providing your body with a continuous supply of vitamin C throughout the day, you are allowing for an extra reserve of the nutrient for your cells to call upon whenever the need arises. This is important for providing the resources to optimize immune function.

Caution:

There is some evidence that individuals who are prone to developing kidney stones should avoid excess vitamin C. Speak with your healthcare provider and always consume fluids throughout the day. Staying well-hydrated is a primary recommendation for preventing kidney stones, according to the National Kidney Foundation.

. . . .

👌 One of the many additional benefits of consuming vitamin C is it supports collagen synthesis, which helps to prevent wrinkles. Who doesn't love an easy and cheap anti-aging solution?

Nutraceutical supplement companies offer the vitamin in a variety of forms: powder, capsule, chewable, buffered and liposomal vitamin C.

There are many good choices to select from. It's best to take one that includes some of the other compounds found in whole foods. Words indicating the other desirable compounds are present include "complex," "antioxidant" or "flavonoids."

Some chewable options contain a lower dose (250 mg), making it easier to take in divided doses. The chewable Vitamin C I recommend may appear to be a children's product, but is used by many adults who want the smaller dose twice daily. Please remember, the recommendations in this book are intended for adults.

When comparing prices on any supplements, check the dosage and see how many servings each bottle contains. Feel free to use information from the labels of products I love to shop around for better deals.

Products I Love

♥ Garden of Life Living Vitamin C Antioxidant Blend, 250 mg

♥ Pioneer Vitamin C, 500 mg

♥ PERQUE Potent C Guard (buffered[37] in powder), 1,584 mg

♥ Natural Factors Big Friends Chewable Vitamin C, 250 mg

♥ Natural Factors C 500 mg, fruit-flavor chew in a peach, passionfruit and mango blend

♥ LivOn Laboratories (Liposomal) Lypo-Spheric Vitamin C 1,000 mg

Caution:

Two potential side effects of supplemental vitamin C are loose stools and stomach irritation. This can be minimized by taking it in divided doses. (Take 250-500 mg at breakfast and then again at dinner.) Or you can further divide the dose between three meals.

If you have a sensitive stomach, choose a "buffered" or "liposomal" form of vitamin C. These forms are more costly, but may be better tolerated. If you still experience any uncomfortable symptoms, back down to the dose you tolerate and try to consume an extra daily serving of a food high in vitamin C.

---

37 Buffered is easier on the stomach.

Vitamin A

VITAMIN A IS NEEDED TO produce important immune compounds. It's especially helpful in fighting respiratory infections, as it reinforces the integrity of your barrier protectors. These barriers are your first line of defense against invading organisms and include the skin and mucous membranes of your nose, throat, trachea, lungs and stomach. Their job is to repel or neutralize foreign invaders, such as viruses. How good are you at keeping unwanted things out?

Vitamin A is just one of the nutrients that augments barrier resistance, making you more resilient right at the initial point of entry for viruses and other invaders.

Because of its essential role in immune resilience, vitamin A supplements of 10,000 to 20,000 IU are often recommended during times of viral exposure or increased immune vulnerability. However, there is some preliminary evidence that supplementing with vitamin A may not be beneficial in all situations. Excessively high levels of supplemental (retinol) vitamin A can also impede vitamin D activity. Therefore, high-dose vitamin A supplementation during a suspected viral infection should only be done under the care of a practitioner who is current on nutritional research.

Food sources of vitamin A are an important part of boosting the immune system all year and especially when you have been in an unhealthy environment. Since this book is primarily focused on prevention, the recommendation is to include foods high in vitamin A several times a week during the year and more frequently during times of increased risk of infection. This is made easier by regularly including dark leafy greens and orange vegetables in your meals. If you eat meat, beef liver tops every item listed below. Sweet potatoes come in close behind. If you're looking for something sweet, pumpkin pie is also a great vitamin A source. Search online for a healthier version of the typical recipe. It doesn't need to be Thanksgiving to enjoy this great American vegetable-based treat.

Food sources of vitamin A include:

Animal Sources

- Beef liver
- Butter
- Cod liver oil

- Eggs
- Salmon
- Shrimp

Plant Sources

- Black-eyed peas
- Broccoli
- Butternut squash
- Cantaloupe
- Carrots
- Collards

- Kale
- Mango
- Pumpkin
- Spinach
- Sweet potato

Minerals

THE MINERALS ZINC, SELENIUM, MAGNESIUM and iodine can be derived from food and a good multivitamin/mineral supplement. You will sometimes find these nutrients included in the combination immune-support products. Some of the elderberry products I recommend contain zinc. And one of my favorite overall immune-support supplements (Source Naturals Wellness Formula[38]) contains vitamins A, C, zinc and selenium.

Zinc

ZINC IS A KEY MINERAL for antiviral immunity and overall robust immune function. It has been the subject of numerous studies. Every component of your immune system is dependent upon zinc. It impedes a virus's ability to attach to cells and replicate once it gains entry. Zinc is involved in the production of immune cells and

---

38 Wellness Formula is by Source Naturals. It is a comprehensive immune formula that contains many of the vitamins, minerals and superfoods mentioned throughout this book, plus additional herbs and propolis (a bee product). Check with your doctor prior to use if allergic to bees.

helps them to maintain surveillance activities. It has proven efficacy in recovery from pneumonia. In addition to evidence showing zinc prevents viral infections, it also reduces the severity and duration of colds and the flu. Moreover, it has been shown to reduce the risk of lower respiratory infection and plays a key role in supporting healthy respiratory function in the elderly and those with compromised lung function.

Zinc deficiency is common, especially in those most at risk for severe infections. In addition to impacting your immune response, zinc deficiency is associated with emotional disorders, poor wound healing, and decreased taste sensation.

Each recommendation in "Multivitamin Supplements" on page 82 contains 15-18 mg of zinc per serving. A multivitamin supplement plus a few servings of high-zinc foods listed here may provide you with the amount you need. If not, you will need a separate zinc supplement. It's challenging to get enough zinc from food alone. The only really good food source is oysters, with 74 mg in three ounces.[39] Beef is next with 7 mg of zinc in three ounces, but beef should be limited for optimal health. The other foods for which we have nutrient data contain much lower levels.

If you inconsistently consume high-zinc foods, consider taking a 15 mg supplement. If you get frequent infections or are in a period of increased susceptibility to infection, consider taking a 25-30 mg supplement to ramp up your body's antiviral immunity. Zinc lozenges are convenient to keep handy for immediate use during times of viral exposure.

I use hemp seeds as a topper for two other high-zinc foods: yogurt and oatmeal. They are also fantastic to use in baking. Garbanzo beans, cashews, fresh green peas, pumpkin seeds and sunflower seeds can also be tossed onto a salad. Remember, you should aim for a large daily salad on most days. Even if you are not accustomed

---

39 According to the National Institute of Health, ods.od.nih.gov/factsheets/Zinc-HealthProfessional/#h3.

to eating them, toss just one half of an oyster into a bowl of clam chowder to ramp up your daily zinc. It won't even be noticed.

· ·

👍 An added benefit of getting extra zinc for those who suffer from cold sores, fever blisters and herpes lesions may be a reduction in the number of outbreaks.

Food sources of zinc include:

- Beef
- Brazil nuts
- Cashews
- Chicken
- Garbanzo beans
- Green peas
- Hemp seeds
- Lamb
- Lentils
- Oatmeal
- Oysters
- Pumpkin seeds
- Scallops
- Shrimp
- Shiitake mushrooms
- Sunflower seeds
- Tofu
- Turkey
- Yogurt

Products I Love

♥ Designs for Health Zinc Supreme, 30 mg
♥ Garden of Life Vitamin Code Raw Zinc, 30 mg

Selenium

THE MINERAL SELENIUM PLAYS A critical role as a defender of the immune systems' white blood cells, which need protection from free radicals. It also plays a supportive role for activating glutathione, a powerhouse antioxidant that is a master player in healthy aging and disease prevention. By protecting white blood cells from free-radical damage produced in their fight against invading organisms, selenium increases the lifespan of critical warrior cells. Benefits of selenium for immune response also include stimulation of antibody production, regulation of inflammation, and the ability to energize the activity of natural killer cells.

Selenium deficiency can cause a virus to mutate into a more serious pathogen. It has also been shown to increase one's susceptibility to diseases associated with aging. A deficiency of selenium makes cells more vulnerable to damage from metabolic compounds, which further impairs immune function.

My favorite way to get adequate selenium is to simply eat one large Brazil nut a day. Sardines are another good choice since they come with the extra benefit of omega-3s, a fatty acid essential for overall wellness. If you are not accustomed to the taste of sardines, try the Spanish-style canned variety. The strong spices help to balance the sardine flavors. Put them on top of a salad for an inexpensive nutrition-packed meal.

Here are some other food sources of selenium:

- Brazil nuts (one a day)
- Beef liver
- Brown rice
- Chia seeds
- Chicken, especially pasture-raised and organic
- Cottage cheese
- Eggs, free-range and organic
- Flaxseeds
- Garlic
- Halibut
- Mushrooms (especially maitake and shiitake)
- Oatmeal
- Salmon
- Sardines
- Shrimp
- Sunflower seeds
- Turkey, especially pasture-raised and organic

Magnesium

The mineral magnesium is involved in managing inflammation and the immune system. Multiple body systems and individual nutrients work together, meaning a weakness in one affects the function of another. Since it is involved in more than 300 enzymatic reactions, adequate magnesium will benefit the entire body.

Magnesium plays a role in activating vitamin D and is involved in multiple immune-activation pathways, including antibody production.

. . . .

👍 Extra benefits of getting adequate magnesium include calming of nervous tension, more restful sleep, and enhanced mood.

Food sources of magnesium include:

🌿 Almonds

🌿 Artichoke

🌿 Banana

🌿 Black beans

🌿 Brown rice

🌿 Buckwheat

🌿 Cashews

🌿 Chia seeds

🌿 Cocoa powder

🌿 Dark chocolate

🌿 Flaxseeds

🌿 Great northern beans

🌿 Kidney beans

🌿 Lima beans

🌿 Molasses

🌿 Mung beans

🌿 Navy beans

🌿 Oatmeal

🌿 Pigeon peas

🌿 Pine nuts

🌿 Potato, baked

🌿 Pumpkin seeds

🌿 Soy milk

🌿 Soybeans

🌿 Spinach

🌿 Squash seeds

🌿 Tahini

🌿 Turkey

🌿 Yogurt

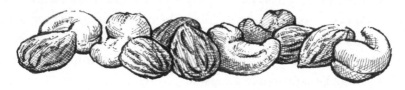

. . . .

👍 There's no need to eat all the foods from each list above. Simply circle foods from each list that you already enjoy. Then circle one more from each list that you are willing to try this week.

Iodine

Iodine is a crucial member of the immune nutrient arsenal for protecting the body from a host of foreign invaders. Experts in this area report most of us are iodine-deficient, which is especially important for people with chronic infections.

Earlier in this book, page 17, I wrote about a seasoning blend with Celtic salt and seaweed. Using this blend regularly provides a good way to get some iodine every day.

My recommendation is to only use iodine supplementation under the guidance of a knowledgeable nutritionist or doctor. Ideally, the dosing is based upon laboratory assessment. Iodine supplementation needs to be done with great care to avoid adverse effects. You can read more about this in the book by David Brownstein, MD, *Iodine: Why You Need It, Why You Can't Live Without It.*

Multivitamin Supplements

Nutrient deficiency is one cause of depressed immunity. Any single nutrient deficiency can weaken the immune system. More is often not better when it comes to keeping your vitamins and minerals in balance. Too much of one can alter the function of another. By following the whole foods, plant-focused way of eating and supplementing your diet wisely, you will get a good balance of most nutrients. A balanced multivitamin supplement is a great way to fill in the gaps.

Since farming soil is often depleted of nutrients, most people still need to take a supplement to fill in the nutrient gaps. These supplements do not in any way replace the bounty of other nutrients in whole foods. Nourishing foods contain life-sustaining bioactives that cannot be captured in a capsule.

To further fine-tune your nutrient balance, you can work with a nutrition practitioner, who can use laboratory testing to assess your exact nutrient needs.

Products I Love

♥   Thorne Basic Nutrients III

♥   Designs for Health Twice Daily Multi

♥   Nature's Way Doctor's Choice 45+ Women

♥   Nature's Way Doctor's Choice 50+ Men

A Friendly Reminder

I know there's a lot of information in here. Please do not feel overwhelmed. We are in this for the long run. Simply choose one new item or habit each week. Start with something easy, so the encouragement from that success will fuel your next step. Do this in a way that's right for you. That's the key to success.

Notice foods that tend to repeat on all the lists above: fruits, vegetables (especially green leafy vegetables), nuts, seeds, beans, lentils, oatmeal, mushrooms, fish and turkey. Let this be a starting place to guide your new meal plan.

Before starting a new nutritional supplement:

○ Check with your pharmacist on any potential drug-nutrient interactions with your medications.

○ Add one new supplement at a time, just to make sure it agrees with you.

○ Understand that nutrient stores can be gently replenished over several months. Taking more than the recommended dosage for an extended period of time can lead to imbalances that disrupt the synergistic teamwork between nutrients and metabolic pathways.

○ Periodically check expiration dates and replace items as needed.

○ If you have an autoimmune condition, your immune system is confused about which cells are healthy parts of your body and which are foreign invaders, so it winds up attacking some healthy cells. In this case, you do not want to overstimulate the immune system. Stay mostly with the food recommendations since they provide more gentle immune support.

○ Be a wise consumer. I have chosen quality brands for product recommendations. When evaluating pricing on alternate brands, check the number of capsules needed to achieve the recommended dose and the total number of capsules in the bottle. You may find less expensive options that require more capsules to achieve the proper dose, which may ultimately be more costly. When unacceptable fillers or inferior ingredients are used, it can make it harder for your body to receive the nutrients it needs. Sometimes fillers are a necessary ingredient in capsules to prevent the clumping of supplements. Cellulose, leucine, rice protein, silica, beeswax, vitamin E, glycerin and sunflower lecithin are among the safer fillers that may be used in small amounts for this purpose.

Chapter 5. Lifestyle Factors That Affect Immune Function

Although this is a short chapter, the importance of its message should not be underestimated. Paying attention to its contents will benefit you in every aspect of your life. Ignoring it will negatively impact your overall health, cause you to age more quickly, increase your risk for brain malfunction, and ambush your immune system. It is so important I can honestly say if you ignore these pearls of wisdom you may not find relief from the antiviral recommendations in the next chapter. That's how important they are. They establish the underlying fabric of your biology.

A landmark 2000 study on lifestyle factors in the Archives of Internal Medicine found smoking and excess weight, along with reduced physical activity, were associated with an increased incidence of pneumonia.[40] This is one of many studies demonstrating the undeniable link between lifestyle and resilience. Sleep, mood and stress management are also among the most well-researched modifiable lifestyle factors that have a profound effect on immune response.

Below you will find healthy living suggestions that have the power to keep your body primed and ready to launch a robust

---

40 Balk I, Curhan GC, Rimin EB, Bendich A, Willett W, Fawzi WW. A Prospective Study of Age and Lifestyle Factors in Relation to Community-Acquired Pneumonia in US Men and Women. *Arch Intern Med*. 2000 Nov 13; 160:3082–88.

immune response in a timely way whenever you need it. These habits will also help to keep your immune cells energized so they stay in the game for as long as needed. Remember, this whole-body TLC will strengthen your resilience in all immune battles, including cancer, diabetes and arthritis, as well as the next flu strain, to name just a few.

Sleep

SLEEP PLAYS A POWERFUL ROLE in supporting healthy immune function. A lack of sleep has been shown in clinical trials to increase the likelihood of developing an infection and, once infected, insufficient sleep will delay your recovery time.

During sleep, your body attends to important housekeeping chores, including maintenance, detox and repair. Sleep is restorative. It's an opportunity for your immune system to reset. Aim for the amount right for your body. For most people, this means sleeping a minimum of seven hours a night and more during times of immune vulnerability.

Have you ever noticed how tired you get when you have an infection? This is your body's signal to return to bed to augment the process of healing. Immune cells require a significant amount of energy to perform efficiently. They can become exhausted as a result of a pathogenic environment, and the ripple effect weakens several aspects of your metabolic machinery. This gives new meaning to the often-ignored recommendation to get more rest during times when you aren't feeling well. It may very well be one of the most important things you do to support and maintain a robust immune response.

The quality of sleep also matters. Here are a few tips to help you have a peaceful restorative sleep:

○ Consider removing electronics from your bedroom, including the television and cell phone.[41]

---

41   Although outside the scope of this book, it should be noted that electromagnetic frequencies have been linked to negative health occurrences, including altered

○ Get some exercise every day. It's a great way to release steam, improve your mood, and prepare your body for rest. Avoid exercising too close to bedtime if you find this overstimulates you and interferes with falling asleep.

○ Avoid coffee, other caffeinated beverages, and chocolate (which contains caffeine) in the late afternoon.

○ Alcohol can initially make you feel sleepy, but then it can disrupt sleep.

○ Shift your brain away from relentless thoughts by recalling two things that happened during the day that you are grateful for. Alternatively, spend your last few minutes of the day praying to shift your brain into a calming gear.

○ Consider experimenting with a weighted blanket if you are plagued by nighttime anxiety.

○ Make your bedroom as dark as possible. Even the light on your alarm clock should be completely dimmed or covered.

○ Keep the room temperature just right; not too warm or cold.

○ Maintain a consistent bedtime and waking schedule.

○ If you need help getting to sleep, try playing soothing nature "music," such as rain or ocean sounds.

○ Avoid eating for at least two hours before bed.

○ Try diffusing lavender essential oil in the bedroom for thirty minutes before bedtime or at the start of bedtime if your diffuser can turn off automatically. Or apply four drops to your hands, rub them together, and then swipe your hands over the pillowcase.

○ Get into bed with an enjoyable book and a low overhead or book light and read yourself to sleep.

○ Sip on a calming tea thirty minutes before bedtime. Here are a few good nighttime blends to make in six ounces of water.

---

immune activity. Three of the simplest things you can do to protect yourself are to never wear a cell phone anywhere on your body, always use the speaker when talking on the phone to create some distance and, when not in use, place the phone at least three feet away from yourself.

Too much fluid and you may be awakened by your bladder in the middle of the night.

Products I Love

♥ Yogi Bedtime

♥ Traditional Medicinals Nighty Night

♥ Twinings Organic Nightly Calm

. . . .

👍 You may discover the wonderful side effect of an improved mood as a result of consistently getting a good night's sleep.

Activity

THERE IS EXTENSIVE RESEARCH SHOWING that regular physical activity enhances the immune response to viral infections.[42] A 2020 study published in the *Journal of the American Medical Association* demonstrated increasing the distance walked each day was significantly associated with lower all-cause mortality.[43]

Physical activity helps the immune system to function at its best by increasing levels of white blood cells. It also prompts the body to increase its circulation of oxygen and nutrients, while decreasing stress hormones. As a result, exercise helps the body to eliminate toxins that can hinder immune activity. When done consistently, it decreases stress and improves mood. Most of the clinical trials showing positive health effects were conducted with aerobic

---

42   Warren KJ, Olson MM, Thompson NJ, Cahill ML, Wyatt TA, Yoon KJ, Loiacono CM, Kohut ML. Exercise Improves Host Response to Influenza Viral Infection in Obese and Non-Obese Mice Through Different Mechanisms. *PLoS One.* 2015 June25; e0129713.

43   Saint-Maurice PF, Troiano RP, Bassett DR Jr, et al. Association of Daily Step Count and Step Intensity with Mortality Among US Adults. *JAMA.* 2020 Mar 24; 323(12):1151–1160.

activities. A systematic review of fifteen studies on yoga found it can be anti-inflammatory and enhance immunity.

Aim for exercising for thirty to sixty minutes daily, but this should be individualized based upon your current fitness level. If you are not accustomed to regular activity, start with just a few minutes. If you are an avid exerciser, be careful to not overdo it; frequent infections may be related to excessive exercise, although consuming nutritional yeast helps minimize that risk.

Choose a time you can be active consistently. The goal here is to keep your body in motion. Add variety to keep it interesting. Avoid overuse of one specific area and allow for flexibility related to timing and weather. A few simple options include walking on a track, walking at the mall (when the weather is not comfortable), and riding a stationary bike at home. You may want to look into a gym or locate organized classes in your community. Staying connected to others is also great for boosting your immune system. Community and group-based fitness classes also help people stay on schedule for going to classes. Babysitting and doing volunteer work are other ways of staying in motion that may be more suitable for you. All movement counts.

If you have any areas of physical vulnerability, focus mostly on activities that do not put too much stress on that part. Swimming is a wonderful exercise for most people who need to avoid straining sensitive body parts. Online classes are available for all levels of fitness, including chair exercises. Divide your exercise into small segments throughout the day if you tire easily with physical exertion.

Mood

EMOTIONS HAVE A TREMENDOUS BEARING on the power of your immune defenses. Your immune system is at its best when you are calm and in a good state of mind. Stress and burning the candle at both ends impair immune function. According to immunologist Rajesh Grover, PhD, "Depression and fear dampen your immune system." Occasional distress is a normal part of life, but chronic distress can alter immune system responses, making you more likely to get sick. If these emotions are chronic, I hope you will seek out a resolution; you deserve to be happy and at peace.

Stress has been shown to negatively alter the bacterial balance in your gut, where most immune activity originates. Negative emotional states and elevated blood sugar increase inflammation, which creates a pathway for viruses to be more harmful. Stress itself leads to increased blood sugar levels. Stress-related eating often includes eating too much sugar and high-carbohydrate snacks, which also leads to elevated blood sugar levels, resulting in elevated inflammation. Supplying your body with healthy foods can reverse this cycle, improve mood, brain health, and immune function.

Controlling inflammation makes following the recommendations in this book even more pertinent. The whole foods and superfoods mentioned earlier will flood your body with anti-inflammatory nutrients and bioactives to combat mood-induced inflammation, especially the colorful vegetables. These nourishing foods and nutrients will also support a more positive emotional state on many biological levels. Pay special attention to getting sufficient zinc and magnesium for additional mood support.

Flavonoid-containing foods, discussed on page 54, have been shown to help regulate emotions as well, including those that remain with us from early childhood. A few common foods with flavonoids include berries, cocoa, green and black tea, fresh parsley, radicchio, cabbage, almonds, pistachios, pecans and olives.

. . . .

☝ Walnuts deserve a special note here. Studies in both animals and humans found they benefit mood, enhance memory, and brain health. The authors of a recent study in the journal *Nutrients*, recommend a handful of walnuts five times weekly.

For a serotonin mood-boosting combo, combine a healthy (not heavy) carbohydrate with a high-tryptophan food. The carbohydrates will help shuttle tryptophan into the brain. Tryptophan is then used as an ingredient to produce mood-boosting, craving-controlling serotonin. Here are a few combinations to experiment with: sweet potatoes and turkey, apple slices with walnuts, or eggs with oatmeal. Need another reason to get moving? Exercise also helps to transport tryptophan into the brain.

Nutrient imbalances further hamper mood management. During times of elevated stress, additional B vitamins are often needed for making neurotransmitters. At the same time, your body may need more vitamin C to support the extra burden on your adrenal glands. This is another reason to make sure you are taking a good multivitamin/mineral supplement every day.

Prescription medications can also deplete specific nutrients. If you are on any medications, ask your pharmacist if any of them are nutrient-depleting. Pharmacists often have a database with information that links directly to your medication list and the related nutrient deficiencies they cause.

Food sensitivities can also trigger brain inflammation, leading to nervous tension and mood disruptions. Remember to consider food sensitivities, especially gluten, as a possible contributor to anxiety, anger and depression.

Consider working with a nutrition-minded practitioner to get professional guidance in bringing your biology, and therefore your mood, into balance. Look for a practitioner who also specializes in gut healing. Many people with mood challenges have an imbalance of gut bacteria or a compromised absorption surface in the digestive tract, known as "leaky gut." This impairs the body's ability to receive nourishment from the foods you are eating. You may be doing a great job with diet and supplements, but if they are only being partially absorbed, you are being short-changed. This gut dysfunction can also have a profound effect on immune function since approximately 70% of your immune system resides in your gut. To locate a practitioner, refer to "Medical Resources" on page 122. Some may even offer phone consultations.

Here are a few simple ideas for enhancing your mood.

○ Avoid overcommitting yourself to the point of anxiety regarding time management.

○ Start each day reflecting on the positive things in your life and your goals. This could also include meditation, prayer or just silent reflection—find what brings you ease.

○ Address emotional toxicity with a professional.

○ Read a book on forgiveness, such as *The Book of Forgiving* by Desmond Tutu.

○ Exercise. It shifts brain function and increases the feel-good neurotransmitter, serotonin.

○ Stay socially connected.[44]

○ Get out in the sunshine and fresh air by taking walks or sit by a window.

○ Swap out the news and violent movies for comedies or comforting forms of entertainment.

○ Find a church that has an organized program of weekly small group meetings for fellowship and study.

○ Spend time pursuing what you are passionate about, such as hobbies, and expressing your creativity.

"Peace, Be Still"

THESE WORDS OF SCRIPTURE WRITTEN around 65 A.D. provide a timely dose of wisdom for life in the twenty-first century. Your mind needs to rest in order to work efficiently. It's important since your mind runs your entire body.

How often do you sit down and do nothing? No cell phone, no television, no music; just sit. Or is your mind running in a continuous loop from one activity to the next worry, and onto another plan? Do you take a sabbath, a day off from your usual chores and tedious

---

44 Volunteering is a great way to meet others, and working together on a common interest creates an immediate bond. Google "volunteer opportunities near me" or go to VolunteerMatch.org to find a situation that appeals to you.

activities? Do you ever just sit in silence outdoors or by a window? If you see a rainbow, do you take time to stop and embrace its beauty?

We are not wired for continuous activity or thought, playing online games, texting, scrolling, talking or watching a screen. Your brain will work better if you give it a rest and not just at bedtime. Consider experimenting with a few minutes of "nothing" time. Sit. Be still. It will help you to become a better version of *you*.

Many people use meditation, sitting outdoors, prayer or short daily devotions to shift into their "Peace, be still" mindset. One book I enjoy using to support this practice is *Jesus Calling* by Sarah Young. Experiment to discover a book or daily practice that works to help you shift into a place of quietness. A refreshed mind will orchestrate the details of your day with clarity and wisdom.

CHAPTER 6. PUTTING IT ALL TOGETHER

Let's start with a quick reminder of what the three phases of immune support are, and then the rest of this chapter will be dedicated to sharing the foods and supplements best used to accomplish each phase's primary goal: keeping you healthy.

- Phase I: Everyday immunity strengthening and care
- Phase II: Exposure to an unhealthy person or environment
- Phase III: Immune-boosting support

Phase I is your strategy for creating a strong immune foundation. Everyday food, nutrient and lifestyle choices will either weaken or strengthen your immune system. This phase consists of overall preventive and strengthening strategies, as discussed in Chapters 1 through 5. It's a program of feeding your cells everything they need to be resilient today, for the next virus[45] that emerges, and as you age. Follow these strategies every day, all year, to the best of your ability.

By contrast, Phases II and III are primarily focused on preventing viral infections and summarize short-term immune-energizing strategies.

Phase II is for times when you are more vulnerable to infection because of exposure to a sick person or an unhealthy environment. The unhealthy environment also includes times when you

---

45   The flu and common cold are respiratory illnesses caused by viruses that can infect the nose, throat and lungs.

are in grief, despair, stress or burning the candle at both ends, just to name a few real-life circumstances that can derail your natural defense system.

Phase III is for times when you are up and about, but feel something coming on. You are not sick yet, but are feeling signs your body requires immune-boosting support. These signs might include an itchy throat, slight congestion or fatigue. These are your body's signals to bring in the reinforcements for a more robust response.

The advice below should be used along with hand washing and other basic safety hygiene practices. These habits will help avoid putting unnecessary stress on your immune system.

These suggestions are preventive strategies to maintain your health by optimizing immune function. They are for non-nursing and non-pregnant adults. They are not treatments for disease. Anyone can sometimes miss the clues indicating they are in Phase II or III. Try to pay attention to the cues your body is giving you at all times. If you wake up feeling sick, consult your primary healthcare provider for recommendations.

The suggestions for Phases II and III are effective *when used immediately*. Timing is everything. It is imperative to equip your kitchen pharmacy now so you are ready for immediate action steps. The whole point here is to use your "weapons" to get ahead of the virus. This means activating your immune soldiers to derail viral activity—all before the virus takes over. That's why timing is crucial.

Everyone is biologically different. Personalized nutrition is the practice of individualizing wellness regimens to match each person's unique biology, health history, emotional, genetic and social needs. It's the wellness map of the future. Since I do not have this information on your current state of health, the general recommendations below may need to be fine-tuned based upon your unique physiology.

The information that follows is meant to serve as a guideline. Since everyone and each circumstance is different, you may need to add or eliminate certain foods and supplements to best address your personal needs. For example, if you are feeling especially vulnerable, you may want more vitamin C. The recommendations are also interchangeable between Phases II and III. If you are in Phase II, but feel you need to be more vigilant in caring for yourself, you can include items from Phase III, such as the Wellness Formula. You may want to do this, for example, when you have been near a sick person and are also under great emotional distress, which diminishes immune function.

The suggestions in Phases II and III will be more effective when you have built a strong foundation through Phase I. Immunity boosting works better when your daily habits (food, mood, exercise, sleep, basic supplements) have been attended to all year long. I understand life gets in the way; you're human, it happens. When you get sidelined, just hop back in as soon as you can. Perfection is not necessary to reap the rewards of building immune resilience.

Note on Vitamin D

If you have been able to follow the monitoring and dosing information from page 66, your vitamin D level should be near the goal of 60 ng/mL. If you haven't, then you are most likely deficient, especially if you don't get out in the sun or if it's winter. If you are in Phase II or III and deficient, take 15,000 IU of vitamin D for three days, then 5,000 IU for three weeks. By this time, you should have been tested and can receive guidance from your practitioner based on your lab results.

Superfoods at a Glance

THESE SUPERFOODS CAN BE ADDED into any phase to help boost your immune system (as well as the other superfoods in Chapter 3).

- Bone broth
- Elderberries
- Fermented vegetables
- Garlic
- Ginger
- Grapefruit seed extract
- Herbs (dried or fresh)
- Immunity teas
- Miso
- Mushrooms
- Nutritional yeast
- Raw honey
- Rosemary
- Turmeric

Note:

All recommendations in Phases I through III
are for daily amounts.

Phase I: Everyday Immunity Strengthening and Care

Objective: Ongoing immune system strengthening,
Timeline: Every day, all year.

Food and Beverage

- ○ Include mostly whole foods.
- ○ Consume five or more servings of vegetables and one to three servings of fruit.
- ○ Include a variety of colors.
- ○ Include a cruciferous vegetable.
- ○ Include adequate protein in each meal along with some snacks.
- ○ Reduce processed foods.
- ○ Cook with generous amounts of herbs and spices.

○ Use ½ teaspoon of nutritional yeast (or the Yeast & Sea Blend).

○ Drink the recommended amount of water or tea throughout the day.

○ Eat one superfood daily.

○ Consume one large or two medium Brazil nuts for selenium.

○ Consume high-magnesium foods.

○ Minimize all the foods and toxins that hinder your immune function.

○ Minimize all toxin-containing food containers, cleaners and personal care products that hinder immune function.

○ Minimize the use of your microwave oven.

Supplements

𝕊 Vitamin D – Get tested two times a year, aiming for 60 ng/mL.

𝕊 Multivitamin/mineral supplement.

𝕊 Vitamin C – 500-1,000 mg daily in divided doses.

𝕊 Zinc – 25-30 mg if you don't get enough from food.

Lifestyle

• **Activity** – Move your body every day for 30-60 minutes. Aerobic exercise, such as walking, is great. Do not overdo exercise, though. It will impair your immunity.

• **Sleep** – Get the amount of sleep right for your body or at least seven hours per night.

• **Mood** – Engage regularly in calming practices and activities that bring you joy. Connect with other people regularly, in any way that fits in with your circumstances.

• **"Peace, be still"** – Make it a priority to have time to be still. If you are not used to this, start with three minutes.

Phase II: Exposure to an Unhealthy Person or Environment

Objective: Activating your immune system.

Timeline: One to seven days after exposure.

Food and Beverage

○ Elderberry – Take according to label directions.

○ Nutritional yeast (or the Yeast & Sea Blend) – Use two teaspoons throughout the day mixed into food.

○ Superfood – Add an extra serving from the list earlier in this chapter.

○ Green tea – Drink two cups with raw honey.

Supplements

⋙ Vitamin C – 2,000 mg daily in divided doses.

⋙ Oil of Oregano – Take one capsule at bedtime. If using oil of oregano drops, follow label directions.

Lifestyle

• **Mood** – Pay special attention to caring for yourself and managing stress by engaging in any practice you find calming.

Phase III: Immune-Boosting Support

Objective: Defending against something coming on.

Timeline: Starting as soon as you feel under the weather, and continuing until two days after you're well again, for a maximum of seven days.

If you are unable to reverse Phase III in three days, consult your doctor for recommendations. Many of the wellness practitioners mentioned in "Medical Resources" on page 122 offer telehealth.

Food and Beverage

- ○ Elderberry – Take according to label directions.
- ○ Vitamin A foods – Consume two servings.
- ○ Garlic – Cook with or consume (in honey) prepared using the Chop & Hold Garlic recipe on page 59.
- ○ Ginger – Cook with generous amounts.
- ○ Juicing – Add a lemon and a small clove of garlic or a small piece of ginger.
- ○ Nutritional yeast (or the Yeast & Sea Blend on page 52) – Use three teaspoons throughout the day mixed into food.
- ○ Soup – Prepare with immune-boosting ingredients, including mushrooms and other superfoods listed earlier in this chapter.
- ○ Green tea – Drink three cups with raw honey.
- ○ Other beverages – Sip broth or other teas throughout the day.
- ○ Minimize sugar and refined carbohydrates.
- ○ Minimize mucus-forming cow dairy (milk, cheese).

Supplements

- ᔰ Vitamin C – 500 mg every two hours (approximately 4,000 mg total for the day)
- ᔰ Oil of Oregano – Take one capsule with breakfast and one with dinner. If using oil of oregano drops, follow label directions.
- ᔰ Wellness Formula[46] (capsules or tablets) – Described in more detail on page 77. Follow label directions under the "Suggested Use" area of the product label.

---

46   Contains a bee product called "propolis." Check with your doctor before taking if you are allergic to bees.

Lifestyle

- **Sleep** – Put aside all unnecessary activity and get extra sleep.
- **Sunshine** – If it's warm, spend fifteen minutes in the sun with your arms exposed (without sunblock).
- **Prevent infection spread** – Isolate yourself, clean shared surfaces, and inform others so they can take precautions (handwashing, wearing masks, and distancing themselves). Let any adults you've been around know to follow Phase II recommendations.

Immunity on a Budget

IN CHAPTER 4, FOOD AND supplement options were provided for each of the key immune nutrients that are commonly deficient in the typical diet. Wherever possible, lower-cost supplement options were offered when I suggested specific products.

My recommendations have been limited to include the most essential foods, beverages and supplements. Even with that streamlining, I recognize the cost of supplements may not be in your budget. Aim to get as many critical nutrients from your food as you can. You spend money on food anyway, so you might as well make sure it delivers all the nourishment you need.

It is possible to get the recommended nutrients through food, especially if you are willing to plan carefully to include an adequate variety of certain foods. Below are recommendations for strengthening your immune system at a lower cost with sunshine, foods that contain key immune-supportive nutrients, soup and spices. These are all great recommendations even if you are using supplements.

Curcumin

- ○ Check out an Indian food blogger to find tasty ways to include the curcumin-containing turmeric or curry spice as a regular part of your menu. Add turmeric to a bottle of salad dressing.

Garlic

○ This is a powerful antimicrobial. Use the chop-and-hold method to ignite its powerful compounds before cooking with it.

Green Tea

○ Consume two to three cups daily.

Herbs and Spices

○ Use all fresh and dried spices liberally. Consider planting rosemary in a pot. It will last into the cool weather; then it can be frozen.

Homemade Tea

○ Consider making a pot of homemade tea by simmering a few slices of fresh ginger in water for five minutes; then add honey and a teaspoon of fresh lemon juice.

Magnesium

○ Consuming seeds, raw nuts, beans and cocoa will help you to get a good amount. Some of my favorite sources of magnesium are pumpkin seeds, almonds and lima beans. The cocoa can be in the form of an ounce of 65% (or higher) dark chocolate or make homemade hot cocoa with one of the recommended sweeteners.

Nutritional Yeast

○ This is effective in small amounts, so you can use just ¼ teaspoon daily.

Selenium

○ Consuming one large Brazil nut a day will provide all the selenium you need. Sardines are another great option—they also supply a good dose of the anti-inflammatory omega-3 fatty acid.

Soup

○ Make a pot of chicken-vegetable or bean-vegetable soup with mushrooms and any other items you like from the superfoods list.

Vitamin A

○ Refer to the list on page 76 and consume these three times a week during the year and every day when you are in Phases II or III.

Vitamin C

○ Refer to the list on page 72 for foods high in vitamin C and use fresh lemon or lime juice in salad dressings, on vegetables, and on any other foods that can use a refreshing flavor lift.

Vitamin D

○ Whenever possible, get most of your vitamin D from sunshine. Expose a good part of your skin (without sunscreen) to noon sunshine for fifteen minutes, three times a week.

Zinc

○ Many people find it's hard to get sufficient amounts of zinc from food when limiting beef to the recommended twice a week or less. Nutrient data reports indicate beef chuck blade roast has more zinc than other cuts, and it's also one of the less expensive options.

○ The only good food source of zinc is oysters, which are not budget-friendly. Since Zinc supplements are fairly inexpensive, they may be the best way to get some of the antiviral nutrient on board.

IF ONE OR TWO SUPPLEMENTS are in your budget, get the Thorne Basic Nutrients III. The dosage of six capsules daily can be divided over six days. It would be better for you to take less of a high-quality comprehensive supplement than to take a poor-quality supplement with questionable ingredient sourcing and fillers. This daily multi-vitamin supplement will help fill in the nutrient gaps in your diet.

The second supplement is Source Naturals Wellness Formula, which is great to keep on hand for when you feel like you are starting to come down with something.

Plan to Saturate

SINCE WE ARE FOCUSING ON creating resilience to prevent anything that may be trying to derail your health, the recommendations throughout the book cover general immune support. If you are serious about seeing the power of natural wellness, you will need a plan. This plan starts with being proactive. Saturate your body every day with an abundance of plant foods that include a variety of colors. You don't need to become a vegetarian. Just make room for plenty of fruits, vegetables, nuts, seeds, legumes and non-gluten whole grains. Concentrate on creating plant-focused meals custom-ized to suit your biology.

For Phases II and III, aim to have the suggested immune-sup-portive compounds coursing through your bloodstream all day; a continuous cocktail to target, engulf and destroy foreign invaders. This concept of saturation is your best bet to send the patho-gens packing.

Taking elderberry at 8 a.m. and doing nothing else to support your system for the rest of the day probably isn't going to work. Remember the juice bathing concept from page 24? It's the same idea here. If you want your immune system to go to bat for you all day long, you'll need to feed it all day. Plan ahead. Stock your kitchen pharmacy. Monitor it regularly for outdated items and restock it as necessary. When the time for extra support arrives, there will be no time for delay!

The Phase II and III recommendations deliver a wide range of dif-ferent bioactives. They are designed to cover all bases as opposed to targeting one specific challenge. Spacing out your immunity-boosting reinforcements, while varying the food and supplement choices, will create the ultimate biological shield to weaponize your body in full armor. Since the body does its best housekeeping (detox, renewal and repair) at night, save one of your supplements for bedtime to make the most of your body's ability to heal itself as you sleep.

CONGRATULATIONS, YOU HAVE MADE IT! My hope is that you now have a good understanding of how to optimize your homeland security system. Please don't wait for a crisis to pay attention to your immune system. The steps taken today will pay off when the next virus hits. These measures will also prep your body for a lifetime of better health. Now is the time to start building resilience by making daily choices to create a strong foundation.

Before we part, I invite you to learn more about my ebook called *Winter Wellness with Essential Oils*. While *Optimizing Your Immune System* has focused on foods and supplementation that support your health, *Winter Wellness with Essential Oils* makes a good companion for those interested in learning more about essential oils. Visit marieruggles.com/winterwellness for more information.

It has been my honor to teach you so you can enjoy the many benefits of proactively boosting your immune system. Remember, health begins when your feet hit the floor every morning. Taking baby steps, building consistent habits, and enjoying some sunshine will bring you to a very good place.

> If you've enjoyed reading this book, please leave a review on your favorite review site. This will help me reach more readers who are interested in optimizing their immunity through building a kitchen pharmacy.

AUTHOR'S NOTE

Thank you for taking the time to read this book and to learn about the care and keeping of your body. Be careful about blindly accepting everything you hear about your health. My hope is that you have been inspired to become an active, educated participant in your care. I encourage you to take back your power by embracing personal responsibility for your health.

Consider praying for clarification and direction regarding advice you receive and for being directed to the right resource (practitioner, online forum, book, etc.). Request that you will be guided to those who are true, wise and the best fit for your personal needs. I have had many health challenges, and this mindset is why I am healthy and able to walk in my purpose today. Don't give your power away. Explore your options.

I believe God has created your body to heal. It just needs prayer first and the proper reinforcements as well. The best reinforcements are those He planted in creation—plants that give us food-as-medicine in many forms, such as berries, spices, teas, herbs and extracts.

In addition to education, part of my ministry is in healing prayer. This book was written under divine guidance, but I can honestly say it pales in comparison to the simple prayer said in faith. Know that you will be in my prayers.

ACKNOWLEDGMENTS

First, I would like to thank Tara Alemany at Emerald Lake Books for her vision, meticulous editorial kraft, and systematic prompts to keep me on track. Right in line with Tara's most recent book, *Publish with Purpose*, she provided the roadmap to delivering meaningful content.

Emerald Lake Books' art director Mark Gerber is the creative talent behind their design work. Mark carefully listened to my ideas and proceeded with a great deal of thought and research. He produced extraordinary images that accurately conveyed my concepts while orchestrating the numerous details of cover design, formatting and layout, often-overlooked features of book design that are so important to a book's esthetics.

Several mentors and colleagues have provided commentary on this book and have also been a source of inspiration. These people are all trailblazers in bringing the science of nutrition into perspective for practitioners who aim to make a difference in the health and lives of others: Diana Noland, John Bagnulo, Kathie Swift, Sheila Dean and Dale Green.

I also want to acknowledge the special role of my content reviewers. They provided much needed practical guidance in clarifying my thoughts and encouragement to get 36,000 words from my head into meaningful sentences. They assisted with manuscript review and provided wise counsel as well: Sabina Fasano, Peggy

Tatalous, Larry Cavagnetto, Julie Mayring, John Fasano, Erik Jakob, Brenda Fulgieri, Maryann Gallucci, Diana Malkin-Washeim, Helen Chasse and Joyce Hummell (my sixth grade teacher who encouraged me to continue writing).

I am deeply grateful to Veronica Anderson, Deirdre Jacobs, Joanne Carrimanico and Susan Young for never tiring of hearing the tedious details of the book's journey, and for their relentless encouragement and prayers.

My gratitude goes out to so many others who have taught me along the way, especially my students, whose enthusiasm for new content has encouraged me to continue extracting the science of nutrition from research into practical steps for everyday wellness.

Immense appreciation is due to the researchers in virology, immunology, microbiology and nutrition, just to name a few. My work is built upon their relentless pursuit of the wisdom of how our bodies work. My gratitude also goes out to the farmers who rise hours before my alarm goes off to care for the plants that are ultimately what brings nourishment to our tables.

Finally, I am indebted to my family who appreciate the lessons on self-care and are (sometimes) willing participants for home experimentation with new concepts and flavors in my exploration of food-as-medicine.

ABOUT THE AUTHOR

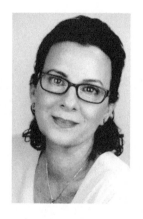

Marie Ruggles, MS, RD, CN, CDE, is a nutritionist and certified diabetes educator and is certified in essential oil safety. She has a master's degree from Columbia University in Nutrition and Public Health where she started her career in research forty years ago.

She then began working in public health, translating the wisdom of science into simple action steps for managing chronic disease and maximizing wellness.

Over time, Marie became concerned about people's lack of reliable information regarding options for being proactive in their own self-care. She decided to write a book that could serve as a home reference guide for her students who were eager to learn about natural options for preventive health and everyday wellness challenges.

Marie is the recipient of national awards for her nutrition education publications and lectures internationally on the safe use of essential oils for everyday wellness challenges.

She is on a mission to inspire others to take responsibility for their personal wellness through nutrition and lifestyle, applying the findings of cutting-edge nutrition research to develop a home inventory of natural wellness options. Marie also advises medical practitioners who are looking to transform their eating habits to align better with the philosophy of their integrative clinical nutrition practices.

When Marie isn't teaching, she enjoys spending time with her family, working in healing prayer ministry, and gardening.

If you're interested in having Marie speak to your group or organization about nutritional support for your immune system, you can contact her at emeraldlakebooks.com/ruggles.

APPENDIX A. MORE ABOUT CRUCIFEROUS VEGETABLES

Consuming a variety of cruciferous vegetables is one of the most important habits to develop for a healthy immune system. They are especially great in helping your body to detoxify and are notable for numerous other health benefits.

I recommend daily consumption of one (or more) cruciferous vegetables or their sprouts with an emphasis on including a green leafy cruciferous vegetable at least three times a week. Many of the green leafy options can easily be included by adding them to a salad.

As for the other cruciferous vegetables, experiment with roasting, which is a flavorful preparation for broccoli, Brussels sprouts, and cauliflower. Roasting brings out the sweetness of vegetables, and you may find yourself devouring this version of a vegetable you previously were not very fond of. Think of these as a daily dose of natural detoxifiers.

Green Leafy

- Arugula
- Broccoli sprouts
- Bok choy
- Broccoli rabe
- Collard greens
- Garden cress
- Kale
- Mustard greens
- Turnip greens
- Watercress

All Others

- Broccoli
- Brussels sprouts
- Cabbage
- Cauliflower
- Horseradish
- Kohlrabi
- Mizuna
- Radish
- Rutabaga
- Turnips

Appendix B. Shopping List

For your convenience, I have pulled together all of the products recommended in the chapters of this book into one quick and easy reference list.

Anthocyanins

- Natural Health Fruit Anthocyanins

Bone Broth

- Kettle & Fire Bone Broth (any variety)

Colostrum

- Natura Health Products Beyond Whey (protein powder)

Curcumin Supplements

- Life Extension Super Bio-Curcumin
- Natura Health Products Botanical Treasures

Elderberry

- Gaia Herbs Black Elderberry (syrup or capsules)
- Gaia Herbs Black Elderberry Extra Strength Immune Support (gummies)
- Gaia Herbs Immune Shine
- Nature's Way Sambucus

Garlic Chopper
- Chef'n Garliczoom

Ghee
- Fourth & Heart

Grapefruit Seed Extract
- NutriBiotic GSE Liquid Concentrate
- Pure Encapsulations Grapefruit Seed Extract

Herbal Supplement
- Source Naturals Wellness Formula

Juicer
- Breville the Juice Fountain Cold XL

Miso
- South River Miso

Multivitamin Supplements
- Designs for Health Twice Daily Multi
- Nature's Way Doctor's Choice 45+ Women
- Nature's Way Doctor's Choice 50+ Men
- Thorne Basic Nutrients III

Mushroom Supplements
- Host Defense MyCommunity (extract or capsules)
- Natura Health Products Mushroom Synergy

Nutritional Yeast
- Foods Alive Nutritional Yeast

Oregano Oil Supplements
- Designs for Health Oil of Oregano
- Garden of Life *mykind* Organics Oil of Oregano Seasonal Drops

Salt

- Premier Research Labs Premier Pink Salt
- Selina Naturally Celtic Sea Salt
- Selina Naturally Celtic Sea Salt Gourmet Seaweed Seasoning

Spices

- Bragg Organic Sprinkle
- Penzeys Turkish Seasoning
- Simply Organic Curry Powder

Sweeteners

All-Natural and Sugar-Free

- Dragon Herbs Sweetfruit Drops
- Lakanto Monk Fruit Sweetener (Golden) with erythritol
- NOW Real Food Organic Monk Fruit Liquid
- So Nourished Monk Fruit Erythritol Blend
- Whole Earth Sweetener Co Stevia Leaf and Monk Fruit

Contains Sugar

- Coombs Family Farms Pure Organic Maple Sugar

Teas

Bedtime Blends

- Traditional Medicinals Nighty Night
- Twinings Organic Nightly Calm
- Yogi Bedtime

Detox Blends

- Choice Reishi Detox
- Mighty Leaf Organic Detox Infusion

Immunity Blends

- Buddha Teas Organic Thyme Leaf
- Gaia Herbs Bronchial Wellness
- Organic India Tulsi Original

- Organic India Tulsi Turmeric Ginger
- Rishi Turmeric Ginger
- Traditional Medicinals Breathe Easy
- Traditional Medicinals Throat Coat (any variety)
- Twinings Organic Peppermint

Vitamin C Supplements

- Garden of Life Living Vitamin C Antioxidant Blend, 250 mg
- LivOn Laboratories (Liposomal) Lypo-Spheric Vitamin C 1,000 mg
- Natural Factors Big Friends Chewable Vitamin C, 250 mg
- Natural Factors C 500 mg, fruit-flavor chew in a peach, passionfruit and mango blend
- PERQUE Potent C Guard (buffered powder), 1,584 mg
- Pioneer Vitamin C, 500 mg

Vitamin D Supplements[47]

Vitamin D with Vitamins K1 and K2

- Designs for Health Vitamin D Supreme with 5,000 IU of D

Vitamin D with Vitamin K2

- Ortho Molecular Products Liquid Vitamin D3 with K2 with 1,000 IU of D
- Seeking Health Vitamin D3 + K2 with 5,000 IU of D

Vitamin D Only

- Carlson Liquid Super Daily D3 drops with 1,000 IU of D
- Nature's Way Vitamin D3 with 2,000 IU of D

Zinc Supplements

- Designs for Health Zinc Supreme, 30 mg
- Garden of Life Vitamin Code Raw Zinc, 30 mg

---

47   Just a reminder. Some companies list vitamin D in micrograms (mcg). For your reference, 25 mcg = 1,000 IU.

Appendix C. Resources

Bonus Materials from the Author

Products I Love

A continuously updated listing, including other favorite immune supplements, foods, spices, kitchen equipment and personal care products. Visit marieruggles.com/products.

Whole Foods Quick Start Guide with Progress Tracker

This is a simple outline to track your progress. It's a summary of all my tips for eating the whole foods way in one place. This will make easy work of implementing changes at your own pace. Download a copy of my progress tracker at marieruggles.com/progress.

Food Resources

Grass-Fed Beef and Poultry

Not all grass-fed practices are equal. Whenever possible, visit the farm or speak with the farmers to learn more about their operation. If you can't do that, explore the websites of these farms.

Below are just a few features to be aware of that will equip you to evaluate the practices of your local farms. It may be too costly for smaller operations to have the features listed below, but they can still offer a good and humane product.

- Provides 100% grass-fed, but if additional feed is required, it's non-GMO.
- Practices regenerative agriculture and soil management.
- Administers gentle on-site slaughter.
- Never introduces antibiotics, growth hormones or steroids.
- Welcomes farm visits.
- Holds ratings or certifications with the Global Animal Partnership, American Grassfed Association, or be Ecological Outcome Verified from Land to Market.

The USDA's definition of "organic" allows for confinement feeding of corn. A good farm will go far beyond the USDA guidelines by allowing their animals to live the most natural life possible. I believe happy livestock make for more nourishing food, and there is actually research to support this.

Concentrated Animal Feeding Operations are thought to be a possible point of origin for the next pandemic since they create the perfect environment for pathogens to be transmitted from livestock to humans. By purchasing healthier, humanely raised grass-fed or pastured livestock, you can have a direct impact on reducing the risk for a serious viral outbreak.

EatWild.com is an international online resource for locating farms that sell grass-fed meat, poultry and dairy products, primarily in the U.S. and Canada, but also in The Bahamas, Malaysia and Panama.

Both of these farms ship to all U.S. states, except Hawaii and Alaska.

- White Oak Pastures: marieruggles.com/whiteoak
- Polyface Farms: marieruggles.com/polyface

Farmers' Markets

SHOPPING AT A FARMERS' MARKET is a great way to try new foods and buy fresh produce while supporting local farmers. Local Harvest will help you locate markets in your area. You can find them at marieruggles.com/localharvest.

Discounted Organic Produce for Home Delivery

THERE ARE SEVERAL COMPANIES PROVIDING discounted organic produce for home delivery. They source fruits and vegetables that are fresh and nutritious, but that would be rejected from the large buyers. Sometimes, it's due to not having a large enough quantity to sell, and other times it's because they are oddly shaped or are too big or small. Search for "discounted organic produce" to see what comes up in your area.

Misfits Market

Misfits Market is a subscription program that sends you quality organic non-GMO fruits and vegetables that are misshapen, over-sized or undersized, making them unsuitable for commercial grocery shelves even though they're perfectly fine for consumption. Even with home delivery, these items are deeply discounted from what you'd find in most stores. Learn more at marieruggles.com/misfitsmarket.

Although this program isn't available in every state yet, there's a waitlist you can join to be notified when they start to deliver in your area.

Online Health Food Stores

THESE RETAILERS FREQUENTLY OFFER SPECIAL promotions and discounts on foods and supplements:

- Vitacost: marieruggles.com/vitacost
- Thrive: marieruggles.com/thrivemarket

Medical Resources

Nutritionists and Natural Medicine Doctors

I RECOMMEND ESTABLISHING A RELATIONSHIP with a nutrition practitioner or a nutrition-minded natural medicine doctor as soon as you are able. This way, if you need help, it will be easier to connect and they will be familiar with your history. Many of them even provide telehealth (phone or computer-based consultations), so you can choose a practitioner from another location.

There are other nutrition and medical organizations that certify nutritionists, herbalists and medical doctors as well. But you can use these organizations to identify the recommended training requirements as a benchmark for evaluating other practitioners you may find.

If you reside outside of the United States, you can locate a naturopathic doctor by searching for your local naturopathic doctor's association or accreditation board.

Integrative and Functional Nutrition Academy

The Integrative and Functional Nutrition Academy (IFNA) maintains an international list of practitioners who are registered dietitians, nutritionists and other healthcare professionals. These individuals have been trained in IFNA's cutting-edge, science-based nutrition program that focuses on identifying root causes and imbalances to significantly improve health outcomes and promote wellness. You can find an affiliated practitioner at marieruggles.com/ifna.

American Association of Naturopathic Physicians

The American Association of Naturopathic Physicians is the professional society representing licensed naturopathic doctors who are trained in accredited medical colleges. They diagnose and treat acute and chronic illnesses by identifying underlying causes and administering personalized treatment plans to address the core imbalances, instead of only addressing symptoms. Naturopathic physicians employ a number of different modalities, including nutrition as well as natural and pharmacologic substances. You can find

122

an affiliated practitioner at marieruggles.com/findadoctor (click "Find a Doctor").

Vitamin D Dose Calculator

THIS CALCULATOR IS PRODUCED BY Grassroots Health, a public health organization dedicated to vitamin D research. Their calculator provides a dosing recommendation for the amount of vitamin D you need to take in addition to your current vitamin D supplement (if you are already supplementing). Enter your weight, current vitamin D (blood level from lab test), and goal vitamin D level into the calculator to get an instant recommendation. You can find the calculator at marieruggles.com/dcalculator.

Laboratory Tests for Inflammation

CHRONIC INFLAMMATION PLAYS A SIGNIFICANT role in most diseases, including cancer. Testing is extremely important since you may not display any obvious signs when you have chronic inflammation. Aim to have these tests taken a minimum of once yearly, but your primary care provider may recommend more frequent testing based on your medical history.

- Hs -CRP (high sensitivity c-reactive protein), which tests total body inflammation.
- Sedimentation rate, which is related to a potential viral infection or autoimmunity.
- Homocysteine, a marker for heart disease, including plaque development and neurological diseases, that is associated with depleted levels of vitamins B6, B12 and folate.

Food Sensitivity Testing

IF YOU HAVE ISSUES WITH food sensitivities, this testing will enable your healthcare practitioner to provide nutrition guidance for foods and food compounds that disrupt your immune system and cause inflammation. Offered by Oxford Biomedical Technologies, the specific test is called LEAP (Lifestyle, Eating And Performance).

For more information contact Oxford Biomedical Technologies at marieruggles.com/leap.

Reading and Other Resources

Newsletters, Magazines and Blogs

TO CONTINUE LEARNING ABOUT SCIENCE-BASED natural wellness, the publications below provide easy reading on a variety of popular wellness topics.

- Johnathan V. Wright, MD, Green Medicine Newsletter: marieruggles.com/greenmedicine
- Metagenics Institute's blog: marieruggles.com/miblog
- Donnie Yance's blog: marieruggles.com/yance
- GreenMedInfo's daily newsletter: marieruggles.com/greenmedinfo

Books

- *The Flavor Bible* by Karen Page and Andrew Dornenburg provides guidance on creating amazing flavor with lists that show which foods and spices go well together.
- *The Microbiome Diet Reset* by Mary Purdy, MS, RDN, is a great resource with recipes for learning more about how to establish a healthy balance of gut bacteria.
- *At Home in the Whole Foods Kitchen* by Amy Chaplin is a vegetarian cookbook that provides guidance on stocking a whole foods pantry.
- *Jesus Calling* by Sarah Young contains brief daily devotions for each day of the year and is useful for your "peace be still" time.
- *The Book of Forgiving* by Desmond Tutu prescribes a path for healing ourselves and our world through the practice of forgiveness.

Healing Prayer Requests, Resources and Training

BRIDGE FOR PEACE (marieruggles.com/bridgeforpeace) is an inter-denominational, worldwide, non-profit ministry. They offer intercession for anyone seeking healing, empowerment and purpose through prayer, scriptural teaching, and resources to support healing prayer training.

STUDY REFERENCES

Age

Balk I, Curhan GC, Rimin EB, Bendich A, Willett W, Fawzi WW. A Prospective Study of Age and Lifestyle Factors in Relation to Community-Acquired Pneumonia in US Men and Women. *Arch Intern Med.* 2000 Nov 13; 160:3082–88.

Diet

Bonaccio M, Pounis G, Cerletti C, et al. Mediterranean diet, dietary polyphenols and low grade inflammation: results from the MOLI-SANI study. *Br J Clin Pharmacol.* 2017; 83(1):107-113.

Burkard M, Leischner C, Lauer UM, Busch C, Venturelli S, Frank J. Dietary flavonoids, and modulation of natural killer cells: implications in malignant and viral diseases. *J Nutr Biochem.* 2017; 46:1-12.

Calatayud FM, Calatayud B, Gallego JG, González-Martín C, Alguacil LF. Effects of Mediterranean diet in patients with recurring colds and frequent complications. *Allergol Immunopathol (Madr).* 2017; 45(5):417-424.

Christ A, Lauterbach M, Latz E. Western diet and the immune system: an inflammatory connection. *Immunity.* 2019; 51(5):794-811.

Handu D, Moloney L, Rozga M, Cheng F. Malnutrition Care during the COVID-19 Pandemic: Considerations for Registered Dietitian Nutritionists Evidence Analysis Center [published online ahead of print, 2020 May 14]. *J Acad Nutr Diet.* 2020; 10.1016/j. jand.2020.05.012.

Iddir M, Brito A, Dingeo G, et al. Strengthening the Immune System and Reducing Inflammation and Oxidative Stress through Diet and Nutrition: Considerations during the COVID-19 Crisis. *Nutrients.* 2020; 12(6):E1562. Published 2020 May 27.

Minich DM, Bland JS. Personalized Lifestyle Medicine: Relevance for Nutrition and Lifestyle Recommendations. *Sci World J.* 2013 Jun 26; PMID 23878520. 186.

Mohammadi Pour P, Fakhri S, Asgary S, Farzaei MH, Echeverría J. The Signaling Pathways, and Therapeutic Targets of Antiviral Agents: Focusing on the Antiviral Approaches and Clinical Perspectives of Anthocyanins in the Management of Viral Diseases. *Front Pharmacol.* 2019; 10:1207. Published 2019 Nov 8.

Molendijk I, van der Marel S, Maljaars PWJ. Towards a food pharmacy: immunologic modulation through diet. *Nutrients.* 2019; 11(6):E1239.

Practice Paper of the American Academy of Nutrition and Dietectics: Nutrition Intervention and Human Immunodeficiency Virus Infection. *J Acad Nutr Diet.* 2018 March; 118(3):486–98.

Spreadbury I. Comparison with ancestral diets suggests dense acellular carbohydrates promote an inflammatory microbiota, and may be the primary dietary cause of leptin resistance and obesity. *Diabetes Metab Syndr Obes.* 2012; 5:175-189.

Wang K, Conlon M, Ren W, Chen BB, Bączek T. Natural Products as Targeted Modulators of the Immune System. *J Immunol Res.* 2018; 2018:7862782. Published 2018 Nov 14.

Wu D, Lewis ED, Pae M, Meydani SN. Nutritional Modulation of Immune Function: Analysis of Evidence, Mechanisms, and Clinical Relevance. *Front Immunol.* 2019; 9:3160. Published 2019 Jan 15.

Young JS. HIV and Medical Nutrition Therapy. *J Am Diet Assoc.* 1997 October; 97 (10 Suppl 2):S161–66.

Yu S, Zhang G, Jin LH. A high-sugar diet affects cellular and humoral immune responses in Drosophila. *Exp Cell Res.* 2018; 368(2):215–224.

Zabetakis I, Lordan R, Norton C, Tsoupras A. COVID-19: The Inflammation Link and the Role of Nutrition in Potential Mitigation. *Nutrients.* 2020; 12(5):E1466. Published 2020 May 19.

Zhi HJ, Zhu HY, Zhang YY, Lu Y, Li H, Chen DF. In vivo effect of quantified flavonoids-enriched extract of Scutellaria baicalensis root on acute lung injury induced by influenza A virus. *Phytomedicine.* 2019; 57:105-116.

Exercise

Bobovcák M, Kuniaková R, Gabriž J, Majtán J. Effect of Pleuran (glucan from Pleurotus ostreatus) supplementation on cellular immune response after intensive exercise in elite athletes. *Appl Physiol Nutr Metab.* 2010; 35(6):755-762.

Nieman DC, Henson DA, McMahon M, et al. Beta-glucan, immune function, and upper respiratory tract infections in athletes. *Med Sci Sports Exerc.* 2008; 40(8):1463-1471.

Saint-Maurice PF, Troiano RP, Bassett DR Jr, et al. Association of Daily Step Count and Step Intensity with Mortality Among US Adults. *JAMA.* 2020 Mar 24; 323(12):1151–1160.

Warren KJ, Olson MM, Thompson NJ, Cahill ML, Wyatt TA, Yoon KJ, Loiacono CM, Kohut ML. Exercise Improves Host Response to

Influenza Viral Infection in Obese and Non-Obese Mice Through Different Mechanisms. *PLoS One.* 2015 June25; e0129713.

Food

Abdullah TH, Kandil O, Elkadi A, Carter J. Garlic revisited: therapeutic for the major diseases of our times. *J Natl Med Assoc.* 1988; 80(4):439-445.

Ankri S, Mirelman D. Antimicrobial properties of allicin from garlic. *Microbes Infect.* 1999; 1(2):125-129.

Barak V, Halperin T, Kalickman I. The Effect of Sambucol, a Black Elderberry-Based, Natural Product, on the Production of Human Cytokines: I. Inflammatory Cytokines, *Eur Cytokine Netw,* 12 (2), 290-6 Apr-Jun 2001.

Castro E, Calder PC, Roche HM. B-1,3/1,6-glucans and immunity: state of the art and future directions. *Mol Nutr Food Res.* Published online March 29, 2020.

Cavagnaro PF, Camargo A, Galmarini CR, Simon PW. Effect of cooking on garlic (Allium sativum L.) antiplatelet activity and thiosulfinates content. *J Agric Food Chem.* 2007; 55(4):1280-1288.

Cavagnaro PF, Galmarini CR. Effect of processing and cooking conditions on onion (Allium cepa L.) induced antiplatelet activity and thiosulfinate content. *J Agric Food Chem.* 2012; 60(35):8731-8737.

Chauhan A, Chauhan V. Beneficial Effects of Walnuts on Cognition and Brain Health. *Nutrients.* 2020; 12(2):550. Published 2020 Feb 20.

Cho SJ, Ryu JH, Surh YJ. Ajoene, a Major Organosulfide Found in Crushed Garlic, Induces NAD(P)H: quinone Oxidoreductase Expression Through Nuclear Factor E2-related Factor-2 Activation in Human Breast Epithelial Cells. *J Cancer Prev.* 2019; 24(2):112-122.

Dai X, Stanilka JM, Rowe CA, et al. Consuming Lentinula edodes (Shiitake) mushrooms daily improves human immunity: a randomized dietary intervention in healthy young adults. *J Am Coll Nutr.* 2015; 34(6):478-487.

Gatti M, Bottari B, Lazzi C, Neviani E, Mucchetti G. Invited review: Microbial evolution in raw-milk, long-ripened cheeses produced using undefined natural whey starters. *J Dairy Sci.* 2014; 97(2):573–591.

Gaullier JM, Sleboda J, Øfjord ES, et al. Supplementation with a soluble B-glucan exported from Shiitake medicinal mushroom, Lentinus edodes (Berk.) singer mycelium: a crossover, placebo-controlled study in healthy elderly. *Int J Med Mushrooms.* 2011; 13(4):319-326.

Gaullier JM, Sleboda J, Øfjord ES. Supplementation with a soluble B-glucan exported from Shiitake medicinal mushroom, Lentinus edodes (Berk.) singer mycelium: a crossover, placebo-controlled study in healthy elderly. *Int J Med Mushrooms.* 2011; 13(4):319-326.

Grimaldi, G., et. al. The potential immunonutritional role of parmigiano reggiano cheese in children with food allergy. *Progress in Nutrition.* 18(1):3-7 · March 2016.

Han F, Ma GQ, Yang M, et al. Chemical composition and antioxidant activities of essential oils from different parts of the oregano. *J Zhejiang Univ Sci B.* 2017; 18(1):79–84.

Hosseini B, Berthon BS, Saedisomeolia A, et al. Effects of fruit and vegetable consumption on inflammatory biomarkers and immune cell populations: a systematic literature review and meta-analysis. *Am J Clin Nutr.* 2018; 108(1):136-155.

Ijaz MK, Chen Z, Raja SS, et al. Antiviral and viricidal activities of oreganol P73-based spice extracts against human coronavirus in vitro. Presented at: Seventeenth International Conference on Antiviral Research; May 2-6, 2004; Tucson, Ariz.

Jesenak M, Urbancikova I, Banovcin P. Respiratory tract infections and the role of biologically active polysaccharides in their management and prevention. Nutrients. 2017; 9(7):E779.

Josling P. Preventing the common cold with a garlic supplement: a double-blind, placebo-controlled survey. *Adv Ther.* 2001; 18(4):189-193.

Kodama N, Komuta K, Nanba H. Effect of Maitake (Grifola frondosa) D-fraction on the activation of NK cells in cancer patients. *J Med Food.* 2003; 6(4):371-377.

Komura M, Suzuki M, Sangsriratanakul N, et al. Inhibitory effect of grapefruit seed extract (GSE) on avian pathogens. *J Vet Med Sci.* 2019; 81(3):466–472.

La Mantia I, Ciprandi G, Varricchio A, Cupido F, Andaloro C. Salso-bromo-iodine thermal water: a nonpharmacological alternative treatment for postnasal drip-related cough in children with upper respiratory tract infections. *J Biol Regul Homeost Agents.* 2018; 32(1 Suppl. 2):41–47. (solution contained GSE; grapefruit seed ex)

Lin WY, Yu YJ, Jinn TR. Evaluation of the virucidal effects of rosmarinic acid against enterovirus 71 infection via in vitro and in vivo study. *Virol J.* 2019; 16(1):94. Published 2019 Jul 31.

Liu JX, Zhang Y, Hu QP, et al. Anti-inflammatory effects of rosmarinic acid-4-O-ß-D-glucoside in reducing acute lung injury in mice infected with influenza virus. *Antiviral Res.* 2017; 144:34–43.

Nantz MP, Rowe CA, Muller CE, Creasy RA, Stanilka JM, Percival SS. Supplementation with aged garlic extract improves both NK and T cell function and reduces the severity of cold and flu symptoms: a randomized, double-blind, placebo-controlled nutrition intervention. *Clin Nutr.* 2012; 31(3):337-344.

Percival SS. Aged garlic extract modifies human immunity. *J Nutr.* 2016; 146(2):433S-436S.

Pilau MR, Alves SH, Weiblen R, Arenhart S, Cueto AP, Lovato LT. Antiviral activity of the Lippia graveolens (Mexican oregano) essential oil and its main compound carvacrol against human and animal viruses. *Braz J Microbiol.* 2011; 42(4):1616–1624.

Porter RS, Bode RF. A Review of the Antiviral Properties of Black Elder (Sambucus nigra L.) Products. *Phytother Res.* 2017 Apr; 31(4):533-554.

Rennard BO, Ertl RF, Gossman GL, Robbins RA, Rennard SI. Chicken soup inhibits neutrophil chemotaxis in vitro. *Chest.* 2000; 118(4):1150–1157.

Saketkhoo K, Januszkiewicz A, Sackner MA. Effects of drinking hot water, cold water, and chicken soup on nasal mucus velocity and nasal airflow resistance. *Chest.* 1978; 74(4):408–410.

Schmitzer V, Veberic R, Slatnar A, and Stampar F. "Elderberry (Sambucus nigra L.) wine: A product rich in health-promoting compounds," *Journal of Agricultural and Food Chemistry.* 58(18) (2010): 10143–46.

Song YJ, Yu HH, Kim YJ, Lee NK, Paik HD. Anti-Biofilm Activity of Grapefruit Seed Extract against Staphylococcus aureus and Escherichia coli. *J Microbiol Biotechnol.* 2019; 29(8):1177–1183.

Summer A, Formaggioni P, Franceschi P, Di Frangia F, Righi F, Malacarne M. Cheese as Functional Food: The Example of Parmigiano Reggiano and Grana Padano. *Food Technol Biotechnol.* 2017; 55(3):277–289.

Thoene M, Dzika E, Gonkowski S, Wojtkiewicz J. Bisphenol S in Food Causes Hormonal and Obesogenic Effects Comparable to or Worse than Bisphenol A: A Literature Review. *Nutrients.* 2020; 12(2):532. Published 2020 Feb 19.

Umesh, Kundu D, Selvaraj C, Singh SK, Dubey VK. Identification of new anti-nCoV drug chemical compounds from Indian spices exploiting SARS-CoV-2 main protease as target [published online ahead of print, 2020 May 2]. *J Biomol Struct Dyn.* 2020; 1-9.

Viapiana A, Wesolowski M. The phenolic contents and antioxidant activities of infusions of Sambucus nigra L. *Plant Foods Hum Nutr.* 2017; 72(1):82-87.

Vinson JA, Cai Y. Nuts, especially walnuts, have both antioxidant quantity and efficacy and exhibit significant potential health benefits. *Food Funct.* 2012; 3(2):134-140.

Zakay-Rones Z, Varsarno N, Zlotnik M, et al. "Inhibition of several strains of influenza virus in vitro and reduction of symptoms by an elderberry extract (Sambucus nigra L.) during an outbreak of influenza B Panama," *Journal of Alternative and Complementary Medicine.* 1 (1995): 361–69.

Zhu F, Du B, Xu B. Anti-inflammatory effects of phytochemicals from fruits, vegetables, and food legumes: a review. *Crit Rev Food Sci Nutr.* 2018; 58(8):1260-1270.

Green Tea

Matsumoto K, Yamada H, Takuma N, Niino H, Sagesaka YM. Effects of green tea catechins and theanine on preventing influenza infection among healthcare workers: a randomized controlled trial. *BMC Complement Altern Med.* 2011; 11:15. Published 2011 Feb 21.

Park M, Yamada H, Matsushita K, et al. Green tea consumption is inversely associated with the incidence of influenza infection among schoolchildren in a tea plantation area of Japan. *J Nutr.* 2011; 141(10):1862-1870.

Steinmann J, Buer J, Pietschmann T, Steinmann E. Anti-infective properties of epigallocatechin-3-gallate (EGCG), a component of green tea. *Br J Pharmacol.* 2013; 168(5):1059-1073.

Minerals

Fawzi WW, Msamariga GI, Spiegelman D, Wei R, Kapiga S, Villamor E, Murakagile D, Mugus F, Hertzmark E, Essex M, Ferencík M, Ebringer L. Modulatory effects of selenium and zinc on the immune system. *Folia Microbiol (Praha)*. 2003; 48(3):417-426.

Guillin OM, Vindry C, Ohlmann T, Chavette L. Selenium, Selenoproteins and Viral Infections. *Nutrients*. 2019 Sept 4; 11(9):15–25.

Gupta S, Read SA, Shackel NA, Hebbard L, George J, Ahlenstiel G. The Role of Micronutrients in the Infection and Subsequent Response to Hepatitis C Virus. *Cell*. 2019 Jun17; 8 (6):120–24.

Haase H, Rink L. Multiple impacts of zinc on immune function. *Metallomics*. 2014; 6(7):1175-1180.

Haase H, Rink L. The immune system and the impact of zinc during aging. *Immunity & Aging*. 2009. 6:9.

Hulisz D. Efficacy of zinc against common cold viruses: an overview. *J Am Pharm Assoc* (2003). 2004; 44(5):594-603.

Prasad AS, Beck FWJ, et al. Zinc supplementation decreases incidence of infections in the elderly: effect of zinc on generation of cytokines and oxidative stress. *Am J Clin Nutr*. 2007. 85:837-844.

Prasad AS. Zinc in human health: effect of zinc on immune cells. *Mol Med*. 2008 May-Jun. 14(5-6):353-7.

Shankar AH, Prasad AS. Zinc and immune function: the biological basis of altered resistance to infection. *Am J Clin Nutr*. 1998 Aug. 68(2 Suppl):447S-4463S.

Singh KP, Zaidi SI, Raisuddin S, Saxena AK, Murthy RC, Ray PK. Effect of Zinc on Immune Functions and Host Resistance Against Infection and Tumor Challenge. *Immunopharmacol Immunotoxicol*. 1992; 14(4);813–40.

Steinbrenner H, Al-Quraishy S, Dkhil MA, Wunderlich F, Sies H. Dietary selenium in adjuvant therapy of viral and bacterial infections. *Adv Nutr.* 2015; 6(1):73-82.

Wong CP, Ho E. Zinc and its role in age-related inflammation and immune dysfunction. *Mol Nutr Food Res.* 2012 Jan. 56(1):77-87.

Multivitamins

Hunter DJ. A Randomized Trial of Multivitamin Supplementation and HIV Disease Progression and Mortality. *N Engl J Med.* 2004 July 7; 351:23–32.

Marston B, DeCock KM. Multivitamins Nutrition and Antiretroviral Therapy for HIV Disease in Africa. *N Engl J Med.* 2004 July 7; 351:78–80.

Rondanelli M, Miccono A, Lamburghini S, et al. Self-care for common colds: the pivotal role of vitamin D, vitamin C, zinc, and echinacea in three main immune interactive clusters. *Evid Based Complement Alternat Med.* 2018; 2018:5813095.

Probiotics

Hao Q, Dong BR, Wu T. Probiotics for preventing acute upper respiratory tract infections. *Cochrane Database Syst Rev.* 2015; (2):CD006895.

Heiman ML, Greenway FL. A healthy gastrointestinal microbiome is dependent on dietary diversity. *Mol Metab.* 2016; 5(5):317-320.

Hojsak I, Abdovi S, Szajewska H, Milosevi M, Krznari Z, Kolacek S. Lactobacillus GG in the prevention of nosocomial gastrointestinal and respiratory tract infections. *Pediatrics.* 2010; 125(5):e1171-e1177.

Wang Y, Li X, Ge T, et al. Probiotics for prevention and treatment of respiratory tract infections in children: a systematic review and meta-analysis of randomized controlled trials. *Medicine (Baltimore)*. 2016; 95(31): e4509.

Quercetin

D'Andrea, G. Quercetin: A flavonol with multifaceted therapeutic application? *Fitoterapia*. 106 (2015) 256-271.

Davis JM, Murphy EA, McClellan JL, Carmichael MD, Gangemi JD. Quercetin reduces susceptibility to influenza infection following stressful exercise. *Am J Physiol Regul Integr Comp Physiol*. 2008; 295(2):R505-R509.

Davis, JM, et. al. Quercetin reduces susceptibility to influenza infection following stressful exercise. *American Journal of Physiology*. August 1, 2008, doi.org/10.1152/ajpregu.90319.2008.

Kaul TN, Middleton E Jr, Ogra PL. Antiviral effect of flavonoids on human viruses. *J Med Virol*. 1985; 15(1):71-79.

Kumar P, Khanna M, Srivastava V, Tyagi YK, Raj HG, Ravi K. Effect of quercetin supplementation on lung antioxidants after experimental influenza virus infection. *Exp Lung Res*. 2005; 31(5):449–459.

Sleep

Besedovsky L, Lange T, Haack M. The sleep-immune crosstalk in health and disease. *Physiol Rev*. 2019; 99(3):1325-1380.

Ibarra-Coronado EG, Pantaleón-Martínez AM, Velazquéz-Moctezuma J, et al. The Bidirectional Relationship between Sleep and Immunity against Infections. *J Immunol Res*. 2015.

Social

Leschak CJ, Eisenberger NI. Two distinct immune pathways linking social relationships with health: inflammatory and antiviral processes. *Psychosom Med.* 2019; 81(8):711-719.

Stress

Agarwal SK, Marshall GD Jr. Stress effects on immunity and its application to clinical immunology. *Clin Exp Allergy.* 2001; 31(1):25-31.

Yaribeygi H, Panahi Y, Sahraei H, Johnston TP, Sahebkar A. The impact of stress on body function: a review. *EXCLI J.* 2017; 16:1057-1072.

Sugar

Della Corte KW, Perrar I, Penczynski KJ, Schwingshackl L, Herder C, Buyken AE. Effect of dietary sugar intake on biomarkers of subclinical inflammation: a systematic review and meta-analysis of intervention studies. *Nutrients.* 2018; 10(5).

Vitamin A

Biesalski HK, Nohr D. Importance of vitamin-A for lung function and development. *Mol Aspects Med.* 2003; 24(6):431-440.

Ross DA. Vitamin A and Public Health: Challenges for the Next Decade. *Proc Nutr Soc.* 1998 Feb; 57(1):159–65.

Vitamin C

Bissell MJ, Hatie C, Farson DA, Schwarz RI, Soo WJ. Ascorbic Acid Inhibits Replication and Infectivity of Avian RNA Tumor Virus. *Proc Natl Acad Sci USA.* 1980 May; 77 (5):2711–75.

Choe JY, Kim SK. Quercetin and Ascorbic Acid Suppress Fructose-Induced NLRP3 Inflammasome Activation by Blocking Intracellular Shuttling of TXNIP in Human Macrophage Cell Lines. *Inflammation*. 2017; 40(3):980-994.

Hemilä H. Vitamin C and infections. *Nutrients*. 2017; 9(4):E339.

Ran L, Zhao W, Wang J, Wang H, Zhao Ye, Tseng Y, Bu H. Extra Dose of Vitamin C Based on a Daily Supplementation Shortens the Common Cold: A Meta-Analysis of 9 Randomized Trials. *Biomed Res Int*. 2018 July 5; e1837634.

Vorilhon P, Arpajou B, Roussel HV, Merlin E, Pereira B, Cabaillot A. Efficacy of Vitamin C for the Prevention and Treatment of Upper Respiratory Tract Infections. A Meta-Analysis in Children. *Eur J Clin Pharmacol*. 2019 March; 75 (3): 303–11.

Vitamin D

Bergman P, Lindh AU, Björkhem-Bergman L, Lindh JD. Vitamin D and respiratory tract infections: a systematic review and meta-analysis of randomized controlled trials. *PLoS One*. 2013; 8(6): e65835.

Cannell JJ, Vieth R, Umhau JC, et al. Epidemic influenza and vitamin D. *Epidemiol Infect*. 2006; 134(6):1129-1140.

Carlberg C. Vitamin D Signaling in the Context of Innate Immunity: Focus on Human Monocytes. *Front Immunol*. 2019; 10:2211. Published 2019 Sep 13.

Grant WB, Lahore H, McDonnell SL, et al. Evidence that Vitamin D Supplementation Could Reduce Risk of Influenza and COVID-19 Infections and Deaths. *Nutrients*. 2020; 12(4):988. Published 2020 Apr 2.

Hossein-nezhad A, Spira A, Holick MF. Influence of vitamin D status and vitamin D3 supplementation on genome wide expression of white blood cells: a randomized double-blind clinical trial. *PLoS One*. 2013; 8(3):e58725.

Martineau AR, Jolliffe DA, Hooper RL, et al. Vitamin D supplementation to prevent acute respiratory tract infections: systematic review and meta-analysis of individual participant data. *BMJ*. 2017; 356:i6583.

Trymoori-Rad M, Shokri F, Salimi V, Marashi SM. The Interplay Between Vitamin D and Viral Infections. *Rev Med Virol*. 2019 March; 29(2):e2032.

Zhou YF, Luo BA, Qin LL. The association between vitamin D deficiency and community-acquired pneumonia: A meta-analysis of observational studies. *Medicine (Baltimore)*. 2019; 98(38):e17252.

Yeast

Auinger A, Riede L, Bothe G, Busch R, Gruenwald J. Yeast (1,3) - (1,6)-beta-glucan helps to maintain the body's defense against pathogens: a double blind, randomized, placebo-controlled, multicentric study in healthy subjects. *Eur J Nutr*. 2013; 52(8):1913-1918.

Fuller R, Moore MV, Lewith G, et al. Yeast-derived B-1,3/1,6 glucan, upper respiratory tract infection and innate immunity in older adults. *Nutrition*. 2017; 39-40:30-35.

Graubaum HJ, Busch R, Stier H, Gruenwald J. A double-blind, randomized, placebo-controlled nutritional study using an insoluble yeast beta-glucan to improve the immune defense system. *Food Nutr Sci*. 2012; 3(6):738-746.

Mah E, Kaden VN, Kelley KM, Liska DJ. Beverage containing dispersible yeast B-glucan decreases cold/flu symptomatic days after intense exercise: a randomized controlled trial. *J Diet Suppl*. 2020; 17(2):200-210.

McFarlin BK, Carpenter KC, Davidson T, McFarlin MA. Baker's yeast beta glucan supplementation increases salivary IgA and decreases cold/flu symptomatic days after intense exercise. *J Diet Suppl.* 2013; 10(3):171-183.

INDEX

cell phones, 87, 92
Celtic salt, 82
cereals, 6, 13, 32
cheese, 13–14, 30, 70, 101
  American, 13–14
  cottage, 80
  goat, 29
  Locatelli, 29
  Parmigiano-Reggiano, 42
  raw, 41
cherries, 73
chia seeds. *See* seeds, chia
chicken, 79–80
  nuggets, 12
  soup, 20, 39, 53–54
chickpeas, 27, 29
chili peppers, 54
chips, 12, 32
chives, 14, 52
chocolate, 87
  dark, 22, 55, 81, 103
  ethical, 22
Chop & Hold garlic, 59, 101
chronic inflammation. *See* inflammation, chronic
cilantro, 21, 26–27, 29, 52
cinnamon, 20, 58
circulation, 33, 88
clam chowder, 79
cleaners, household, 3, 99
cloves, 55, 58
cocoa, 22–23, 35, 81, 90, 103
coconut milk. *See* milk, coconut
coconut oil. *See* oils, coconut
coconuts, 15, 33, 41, 46
coconut water, 62
cod liver oil. *See* oils, cod liver
coffee, 23, 87
colds, 78

collagen, 70, 74
collard greens, 18, 70, 113
collards, 77
colostrum, 49
compounds
  anti-inflammatory, 72
  cancer-preventive, 72
  immune, 76
  metabolic, 80
congestion, 4, 44, 96
containers, 4, 9, 35, 99
  glass, 15, 35
  plastic, 54
convenience foods, 3, 8–11, 35, 42, 64
  containers for, 9
  minimally processed, 14
  organic, 6
  reducing, 12, 98
  toxins in, 4
cookware, 35
corn, 13–14, 28–29
corn syrup, 12
cosmetics, 5
cottage cheese. *See* cheese, cottage
cranberries, 28
cress, 27, 29
  garden, 113
cruciferous vegetables, 18, 34–35, 40, 98, 113
cucumbers, 25–28
curcumin, 47–48, 102
curry, 47–49, 102

D
dairy, 29–30, 33, 41, 49
  cow, 101
  excess, 35
deli meats, 12
depression, 89, 91

For more great books, please visit
emeraldlakebooks.com.

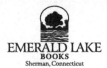

EMERALD LAKE
BOOKS
Sherman, Connecticut